COCAINE HANDBOOK

Now that it has come into everyday use, however, it is important that its chemical reactions should be as well known as those of quinine or caffeine, since it is now liable to come under observation in medico-legal investigations. It is also desirable that the physical properties of cocaine salts should be familiar, so that purchasers may be on their guard against substitutions or adulterations.

NOTES ON THE ALKALOIDS OF COCA LEAVES

A. B. Lyons, M.D.

The American Journal of Pharmacy.

OCTOBER, 1885

COCAINE HANDBOOK

AN ESSENTIAL REFERENCE

David Lee

Printed in the United States of America

First Printing: October 1981

10 9 8 7 6 5 4 3 2 1

The author's gratitude must be expressed to the people at And/Or Press whose efforts, professional expertise and moral support have transformed a handful of typewritten pages into a thing of beauty.

Project Director: Sebastian Orfali
Developmental and Manuscript Editor: Nicholas Flamel
Copy Editor: Jim Schreiber
Appendix Research: Bebe Bertolét
Cover Design and Art Direction: Carlene Schnabel
Book Design: Carlene Schnabel, Suellen Ehnebuske, Marlyn Amann
Diagrams: Phil Gardner, Carlene Schnabel, Nicholas Flamel
Chart Design & Format: Marti Craig of PrePrint
Pasteup: Marlyn Amann, Marian O'Brien, Phil Gardner, Sally Taback, Catherine Conner
Typography: Accent & Alphabet, Marti Craig of PrePrint, Aurora Typesetters
Cover Typography: Petrographics, Aurora Typesetters
Proofreading: Martha Benson, Sayre Van Young, Jean Haseltine, Bebe Bertolét
Index: Sayre Van Young

Library of Congress Cataloging in Publication Data

Lee, David, 1944 Sept. 22–1980 Jan. 12
Cocaine handbook.

Bibliography: p.
Includes index.
1. Cocaine habit. 2. Cocaine. I. Title.
HV5810.L44 362.2'93 81-10865
ISBN 0-915904-56-X AACR2

The publisher would like to thank the following for their permission to use these materials:

p. 7: Introduction, copyright © 1981 by Michael Aldrich.

p. 43: Photo reproduced courtesy of Wide World Photos.

p. 49: Comic strip, copyright © 1977 by Gilbert Shelton and Dave Sheridan; from *The Adventures of Fat Freddy's Cat;* published by Rip Off Press, Inc., San Francisco.

p. 54: Tips on Health Care, copyright © 1981 by Michael Aldrich.

p. 58: Doonesbury comic strip, copyright © 1980, G.B. Trudeau. Reprinted with permission of Universal Press Syndicate. All rights reserved.

p. 56: Coke & Sex, copyright © 1981 by Michael Aldrich.

p. 57: Treatment of Cocaine Overdose, copyright © 1981 by Michael Aldrich.

p. 59: Dr. McDope's Amazing Facts cartoon, copyright © 1980 by R. Siegel, D. Sheridan, and P. Ryan. Used with permission.

In addition, we gratefully acknowledge the numerous contributions by the individuals whose work is cited below the brief quotes used for reference throughout this work.

Neither the author nor the publishers condone or encourage the possession, use, or manufacture of any illegal substances. The material herein is presented for reference and informational purposes only. The author and publisher advise against any application of the procedures herein if they involve breaking the law or any hazard to persons and/or property. Some of the procedures documented, especially those involving volatile solvents or concentrated acids and alkalis may be extremely hazardous. The reader is cautioned not to perform any of these procedures. The procedures described should only be performed under laboratory conditions by professional chemists operating under the authority of the proper government regulatory agencies.

Sometimes we are attracted
to things we must avoid.
Some things in life cannot be explained,
without being destroyed.
I can see it when you look at me,
I can feel it deep inside;
You've moved me in a hundred ways.
It cannot be denied.
When it's time for me to go,
it won't be of my choosing.
Even though the world seems made
of winning, and of losing;
There is a price I will not pay.
A price I'll be refusing.

—David Lee
9/22/44 - 1/12/80

TABLE OF CONTENTS

Introduction by Michael Aldrich 11

Author's Preface 17

CHAPTER ONE:
Mama Coca 23

CHAPTER TWO:
The Alkaloids 32

CHAPTER THREE:
Understanding the Cocaine Trade 40

CHAPTER FOUR:
The High Cost of Getting High 47
- Cocaine and Health 47
- Cocaine and Economics 62
- Cocaine and the Law 63

CHAPTER FIVE:
Adulterants 70

CHAPTER SIX:
Testing 76
- On Location: 77
  - Sensory Tests; Methyl Benzoate; Solubility; Clorox II; Foil Burn
- At Home: 101
  - Melting Point; Cocaine Base Test
- In the Lab 123

Color Plates 127

CHAPTER SEVEN:
Purification 146
- The Acetone Wash 147
- Crystallization: 155
  - Crystal Growth; The Chemicals; The Solvents; The Acid; Stirring; When Is Crystallization Complete?; Washing the Crystals; Drying the Crystals

Appendix A: DISCONTINUING COCAINE ABUSE 173

Appendix B: LABS 175

Appendix C: HEALTH CENTERS 179

Glossary 191

Bibliography 195

Index 197

BLACK & WHITE PHOTOGRAPHS

PHOTOS 1-4:
Pieces and Duff 81-82
PHOTOS 5-24:
Microphotos of Cocaine and Adulterants 83-86
PHOTOS 25-27:
Solubility Test 88
PHOTOS 28-62:
Clorox Test 91-99
PHOTOS 63-64:
Foil Burn Test 102-103
PHOTOS 65-69
Melting Point Test 105-109
PHOTOS 70-94:
Cocaine Base Test 111-122
PHOTO 95:
pH Test Paper 123
PHOTOS 96-109:
Acetone Wash 148-152
PHOTOS 110-136:
Crystallization 158-168

COLOR PLATES

PLATES 1-6:
Coca Plant and Leaves 129-131
PLATES 7-32:
Cocaine in Various Forms 132-141
PLATES 33-56:
Results of Melting Point Tests 142-143
PLATES 57-68:
Results of Foil Burn Tests 144

CHARTS, DIAGRAMS, AND BOXES

CHART:
Summary of Purity Tests for Cocaine with Common Adulterants (inside front cover)
BOX:
Vin Mariani Testimonials 26
BOX:
Essentials for Cultivation of Coca 28
CHART:
Species of Coca and Their Characteristics 30
DIAGRAM:
The Cocaine Molecule—Its Structure and Its Decomposition 34
CHART:
Primary Coca Alkaloids and Their Properties 38
DIAGRAM:
Cocaine Trade Hierarchy from Farm to Consumer 45
CHART:
Treatment for Cocaine Reactions—A Summary 51
DIAGRAM:
Damage to the Nose Must be Mended Surgically 53
BOX:
Tips on Health Care 54
BOX:
Coke & Sex 56
BOX:
Treatment of Cocaine Overdose 57
BOX:
Two Opinions 61
CHART:
An Overview of Cocaine Laws and Penalties for the 50 States 64
CHART:
Adulterants Found in Cocaine—Frequency of Appearance 73
CHART:
Solubilities of Cocaine and Common Adulterants 89
CHART:
Melting Points of Cocaine and Common Adulterants 107
CHART:
Cocaine Base Test: Problems and Remedies 113
DIAGRAM:
Cocaine Solubility—In Acidic and Basic Solutions 154
CHART:
Crystallization of Cocaine Hydrochloride: Problems and Remedies 156

INTRODUCTION

by Michael R. Aldrich, Ph.D.

> The life of a drug taker can be a happy one, or it can be one of suffering and misery: it depends on the user's knowledge.
>
> James Lee,
> *Underworld of the East,* 1935.

Cocaine is a dangerous drug. It is not marijuana. Cocaine has its own karma of mental and physical effects: improperly used, it can lead to severe nose, heart, and respiratory problems. It can cause sudden death. Whether these sobering realities occur or not is up to the user. The drug itself can't decide whether it will be used well or badly, and the drug doesn't care.

Moreover, cocaine is perhaps the most "positively reinforcing" of drugs. Lab monkeys will kill themselves trying to get it. The difference between a monkey and a human in this regard is that the human can be very discriminating about what gets put into his or her system. First by asking questions, then by making subtle distinctions and choices, the human can become a connoisseur.

Connoisseurship means paying attention. Connoisseurship is a yoga of personal health care, will power, and moral responsibility. This is more than just status-seeking, and much more than the ability to identify different products or perform simple tests of product purity. Ultimately, connoisseurship means saving your own life.

The purpose of this book is consumer protection, which begins with quality control. In 1978, the U.S. government estimated that 6.5 million Americans had tried cocaine, and that number has probably tripled by now. But most consumers have never seen real cocaine.

Pure cocaine is the Holy Grail. It sparkles like the snow. It goes in easy in the nose. It doesn't burn. Soon you feel no pain. That's sweet cocaine.

Pure cocaine, in its water-soluble hydrochloride (salt) form, is much easier on the nose than the adulterants, other coca alkaloids, and residues of acids and solvents that usually accompany it in the illicit market. To begin the process of caring for your only nose, search for the pedigree: a lineage of growers, refiners, importers, and dealers who would rather raise the price than cut the product. Unfortunately, such a pedigree is very hard to find. Even dealers cannot often get unadulterated cocaine. So finally, even in the best of worlds, the consumer is on his own. Hence the need for this book.

Alchemy lives! In this audaceous new volume, David Lee has corrected, revised, and added much new information to his *Cocaine Consumer's Handbook* (And/Or Press, 1976). David devoted the last three years of his life to checking and re-checking these procedures, and died of cancer before the new edition went to press. Because of his efforts, the secrets of cocaine alchemy are now revealed for the first time in public print. How to test a sample for adulterants and impurities; how to remove them; how to transform street grit into pearl. Such detailed technical information is the *sine qua non* of cocaine connoisseurship, and is David Lee's legacy to the world.

However, the warning at the beginning of this book is no joke: all procedures involving flammable substances, especially volatile solvents like ether and acetone, should be done only by a skilled chemist in a real laboratory. The finest, purest cocaine is worthless if you're not around to enjoy it.

Understanding the alchemy that produces cocaine is just the beginning of connoisseurship. Ironically, most consumers don't like pure cocaine — it's "too strong" and causes teeth-grinding wiredness unless incredibly small doses are used. The ideal natural dose of cocaine is that delivered by chewing coca leaves — a tiny amount released slowly and steadily into the system along with a nice complement of vitamins and minerals. If someone is not getting off on one or two half-inch (5 milligram) lines, the coke is cut and sniffing more simply means sniffing more cut. With uncut cocaine, the optimal dose is at least half and perhaps one-fourth the size of a usual line. In these circumstances, laying out tiny little lines is a source of pride, not of embarrassment. It says, in effect, that it's the real thing.

The key to successful cocaine use is to USE IT LESS THAN YOU WANT TO. Put another way, "moderation in all things" is the way to protect oneself against cocaine abuse. This takes real will power, which begins by turning down a pretty white powder when one knows it's been cut to smithereens, and by using uncut cocaine unbelievably sparingly. Eventually, as David Lee points out, if consumers refuse to buy or use adulterated cocaine, dealers will be forced to offer a cleaner product. Connoisseurship is the only real leverage a consumer has in the illicit market. If enough consumers become connoisseurs and maintain high standards of quality in their purchases, this will ripple all the way back through the market to South American cocales and refineries where cocaine is first manufactured.

The natives of Andean America long ago discovered that cocaine (in coca) is helpful when working or traveling at high altitudes where oxygen pressure is low. In tiny doses, it stimulates the central nervous system, especially the electrical activity of the brain and the cardiovascular and respiratory systems, without damaging bodily tissues.* It increases the metabolism enough to ward off the extreme exhaustion and nausea (mountain sickness) that people feel when deprived of oxygen. When pure cocaine hydrochloride, instead of coca, is used at altitudes below about 12,000 feet, the drug instantly boosts all bodily systems just as it would at high altitude. This is the source

---

* See S. J. Mulé, ed., *Cocaine: Chemical, Biological, Clinical, Social and Treatment Aspects,* CRC Press, Cleveland, 1976.

of the euphoria and increased vigor that users desire.

This additional energy is rarely expended by contemporary cocainists who use it as a party drug rather than a work drug. Here the energy is cycled even faster with big doses repeated fairly frequently. It builds up rapidly until it peaks, which is the state sought by users. After that the energy drains away until the consumer has a strong urge—sometimes an "uncontrollable" craving—for another hit. This mini-cycle of reward and sag, reward and sag, constantly reinforces the user's desire for more. "Psychological dependency" is the moral trick, the sudden curve at the end of the tunnel of rewards. Self control is the only way to break the cycle. The ability to say NO is the mark of the real connoisseur.

In the excitement of sweet cocaine, people tend to ignore the signals of stress that their body is giving them. The reward-and-sag cycle leads to increased doses and more frequent use of the drug. Tolerance builds up. To recapture the unique grace of a first hit, users snort more and more, or turn to injecting it or smoking freebase. When the party's over and they can't get to sleep, they drink alcohol, take a downer, or smoke a lot of weed. In the morning they feel utterly crummy, and reach for another hit to start the cycle again.

If cocaine is used in this manner for days, weeks, or months, all the systems involved in the energy boost are severely stressed and often damaged. The chronic coke sniffer is an easy prey for bacterial infections in the nose and throat because the proper flow of mucus on these vital membranes is disrupted. Cocaine is a strong vasoconstrictor: it constricts the blood vessels which supply oxygen to living tissues such as the septum. This causes an ulcer which may wear right through and perforate the cartilage. Not just cuts, but cocaine itself damages the nose when snorted: lidocaine, procaine, and caffeine are even worse.

Moreover, the cardiovascular system is stressed and may suddenly malfunction, causing a heart attack. Smoking freebase is especially dangerous in this respect. Cocaine increases the heart rate and blood pressure, so people with heart problems or high blood pressure should not use cocaine at all. Finally, cocaine acts locally as an anesthetic by blocking nerve transmission, and simultaneously overstimulates the sympathetic nervous system; synaptic messages get garbled or not sent, resulting in anxiety, paranoia, poor judgment, and tactile or auditory (rarely visual) hallucinations. While the brain is frenzied, the nerves and muscles controlling the heart and lungs may be anesthetized and these vital organs simply stop functioning. In an overdose situation, which usually happens so fast that nothing can be done about it at home, delirium, respiratory depression, gasping for air, convulsions, and unconsciousness followed by death from respiratory failure may result. This is the wrong way to use cocaine.

A less harmful way for the consumer to use cocaine is to pay close attention to his body and mind, his pocketbook and his product. Real cocaine is preferable to cuts. The user should buy less than he can afford. If there is any reason to suspect that coke is not pure, it can be tested or sent to a lab. Drug Enforcement Administration rules prevent drug analysis labs from revealing the percentage of purity of a sample, but they can state what other chemicals are in it. Impurities can be removed first; then the cocaine can be diluted with a relatively harmless adulterant like mannitol. At least the user will then know exactly what he's putting into his system.

Don't snort freebase — it's not water soluble and will just act like a clod of dirt in your nose. I share David Lee's aversion to freebase smoking and don't recommend it to anybody. Though the first hit can be quite a rush, that feeling is impossible to recapture in succeeding hits, and the danger of overdose is ever-present. The same applies to injecting it. Injecting street cocaine is absolutely crazy — imagine putting quinine, talcum powder, or borax in your heart and brain. Smoking freebase is as dangerous as injecting the hydrochloride. A substance when smoked enters the brain more rapidly than an injected substance; and the blood flow dilutes an injected dose as it circulates, while a smoked dose is less diluted. Smoking freebase and injecting the hydrochloride are the worst alternatives to snorting in terms of health. A user whose nose is worn out can switch to tooting under the tongue or dissolving a pinch of coke (0.05–0.10 gram) in a glass of wine and drinking it. Though the effects of oral ingestion are somewhat different, the high can be quite superior.

When working behind cocaine, connoisseurs do it no more than three times a day, to build up a gentle plateau of stimulation like that provided by coca. Personally, I find a cup of coffee in the morning and another in the early afternoon a much better stimulus for work.

Connoisseurs who party with cocaine treat it like a guest — a temporary visitor, not a resident. They become consciously aware of how much it takes to get them high — this varies with individuals — and stop there. They recognize the excitement of sweet cocaine and take it easy. They aren't greedy, and don't show off about how much they can toot. Soon they'll discover what level is optimum for them, and how to maintain that level with progressively smaller, not larger, doses. They set a time limit: "Okay, I'm going to get high until midnight, but that's enough. There's always a next time."

Temporary abstinence greatly increases the power of the next high. Between parties, connoisseurs go without cocaine, and space coke sessions well apart. They pay attention to that feeling of revulsion for cocaine that chronic users often get: it means it's time to stop using coke for a while. Only if the lag is present can the body and mind restore themselves to normal health; and only then is the reward worthwhile. Connoisseurs go easy and live.

Michael R. Aldrich, Ph.D.

San Francisco
October 1980

AUTHOR'S PREFACE

When the *Cocaine Consumer's Handbook* was first written, in the fall of 1975, I firmly believed that the cocaine market had peaked. More and more, independent entrepreneurs were being squeezed out of the cocaine black market by larger organizations whose widening control soon extended from the coca fields of South America to the streets of many United States cities. As with any monopoly, the result of the illicit cocaine trade being channeled through a few large organizations (instead of many small-time operators) was a radical drop in quality accompanied by a steep climb in price. Whereas high quality cocaine was at one time available to the consumer, the illicit market has deteriorated to the point where the consumer is fortunate if what he buys is 50% cocaine.

The dangers of this market condition are quite obvious. If cocaine ingested by the consumer is less than 50% pure, what else is he consuming? When the consumer could obtain high quality illicit cocaine, he could be reasonably certain how he would be affected and of the risks involved in ingesting this illegal substance. However, when the cocaine has been adulterated, it becomes increasingly difficult for the consumer to be aware of what risks may be involved. In addition, he has been defrauded of his money. What is the consumer to do?

A parallel exists between the state of the present cocaine market and the marijuana market of the late 1960s and '70s which may provide some insight into the problems and a clue to a possible solution. In the 1960s marijuana was available from several foreign sources. The quality was high and the prices were low. As the demand began to exceed the supply, importing larger amounts of marijuana became necessary. The emphasis rapidly shifted from quality to quantity in order to meet the demand. In 1969, Operation Intercept, later called Operation Cooperation, was instituted between the United States and Mexico. This attempt to curb the flow of illegal marijuana between these two countries was a prime factor in putting the small-time smuggler out of business. The larger organizations had means of avoiding the legal problems and were soon in total control of the market. Marijuana had become big business, and as long as it continued to sell there was little reason to be concerned with trivial matters such as quality or the health hazards caused by herbicides like Paraquat. The consumers' only recourse was to refrain from using marijuana, and, though some did, the majority of people accepted the change. It was a sellers' market, at the consumers' expense.

At about this time, small amounts of domestically grown marijuana were available, but were considered inferior in quality. A few pioneering cultivators, mostly in Hawaii and California, developed strains of marijuana which rivaled or even surpassed the finest foreign strains. As consumer awareness increased, homegrown rapidly changed from a dirty word to a preference. Across the United States, inspired consumers of marijuana began cultivating their own strains. The U.S. cultivator became an important source of illegal marijuana, and today it is the foreign varieties which meet with market apathy and skepticism.

While it is virtually impossible for U.S. cultivators to grow enough coca to produce enough cocaine to meet the demand, the consumer still has the power to force the cocaine black market to raise the quality. Since the suppliers of illicit cocaine have not taken it upon themselves to provide an unadulterated, properly refined product, the consumer must set his own standards for quality and reject those products which do not meet these standards. Many consumers are already learning how to avoid adulterated cocaine and are using simple techniques to remove adulterants which are present or further refine a crude product. In this way, the informed consumer has an alternative to inferior quality cocaine. Only through alternatives will the the consumer have the means and desire to say no to unscrupulous dealers who continue to sell a product no matter what its contents may be. As more and more adulterated cocaine is rejected at the marketplace, the suppliers will be forced to provide a saleable product. This book is dedicated to providing the information which is necessary to give the consumer these alternatives. It is my hope that a free flow of truthful information can and will restore some semblance of integrity to a market rarely noted for these qualities.

January 1980

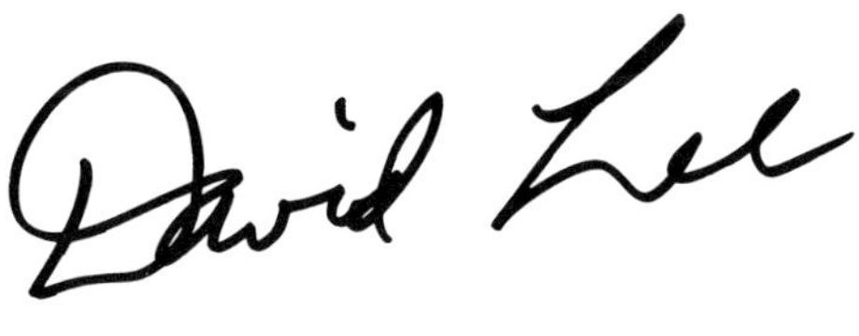

COCAINE HANDBOOK

An Essential Reference

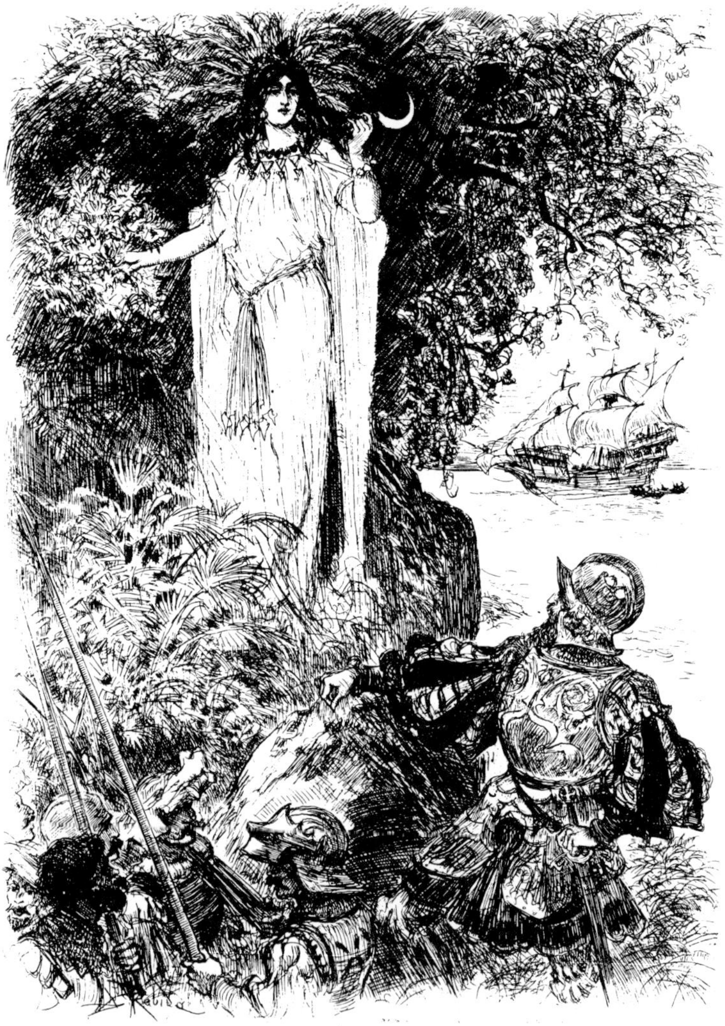

Mamma Coca Presenting the "Divine Plant" to the Old World [Etching by Robida from the 1904 French Edition of W. G. Mortimer's *History of Coca*].

Chapter One

Mama Coca

. . . coca is an integral part of the Indians' way of life, deeply involved with his traditions, his religion, his work and his medicine. To deny the use of coca to the Indians is as serious a disregard for human rights as would be an attempt to outlaw beer in Germany, coffee in the Near East or betel chewing in India. The recent attempts to suppress and control the use of coca can be interpreted only as the latest step in the white man's attempt to exterminate the Indian way of life and make him completely dependent on the alien society and economy which has gradually surrounded him.

Richard T. Martin,
Economic Botany, 1970.

Coca is not cocaine. For centuries prior to the isolation of cocaine as coca's most active ingredient, the Indians who lived on the eastern slopes of the Andes in Bolivia and Peru chewed the leaves as a way of life. Their knowledge of the plant's virtues was passed on from generation to generation by wad of mouth.

Coca is consumed by chewing the leaves with a pinch of lime prepared from calcinated seashells or plant ashes. Prior to adding the lime, the leaves are chewed to moisten and break them, as well as remove the stalks and strings. Then the lime is added pinch by pinch until the proper mixture is achieved. The wad of leaves is then kept relatively still between the teeth and cheek; it is sucked on rather than chewed. The amount of lime used is critical to the taste and to the concentration of alkaloid released. It is still a common practice for a mother to introduce her young to the coca experience by preparing the wad of leaves in her mouth and then transferring it to the mouth of her child. In this way, the proper amount of lime will be present in the first wad of leaves the child uses, which ensures that the first experience with coca will be a positive

"...certain coqueros, eighty years of age and over, and yet capable of such prowess as young men in the prime of life would be proud of."

Dr. Hipólito Unanue, 1794, commenting on the aphrodisiac value of the coca plant (in R. T. Martin, 1970).

one. Since lime is caustic, an excess will burn the mouth. Without any formal knowledge of chemistry, these Indians were extracting the alkaloids from the leaves by making them alkaline. They knew that the lime was the mechanism by which absorption of the alkaloids could be controlled. Thus, if while chewing the leaves a little too much alkaloid was released, one had only to ease up on the lime and let the saliva wash out some of the excess lime into the stomach. The lower concentration of lime would result in a slower absorption of alkaloids. Interestingly, cocaine alkaloid content was not the prime factor in choice of leaves. The Indians consistently chose leaves with a lower cocaine content but a high concentration of sweet, aromatic compounds which gave the wad of coca better flavor.

Over the years South American Indians have found the leaf beneficial in numerous ways. Aside from its ability to clear the mind, elevate mood, and make energy available, it appears to exert good influences on many physical functions. For example, it tones and strengthens the entire digestive tract, probably enhancing the assimilation of foods. A hot water infusion of coca sweetened with a little raw sugar (called *agua de coca*) is an excellent remedy for indigestion and stomach ache that was widely used even by non-Indians throughout South America until relatively recently.

> Coca appears to maintain the teeth and gums in a good state of health; it keeps teeth white. The leaf is rich in vitamins, particularly thiamine, riboflavin, and C. An average daily dose of coca leaves (two ounces) supplies an Indian of the High Sierra with much of his daily vitamin requirement. Coca appears to have a beneficial influence on respiration, and is said to effect rapid cures of altitude sickness. It also rids the blood of toxic metabolites, especially uric acid. Indians say that regular use of coca promotes longevity as well. According to Indian tradition, coca was a gift from heaven to better the lives of people on earth.
>
> (From Andrew Weil's "The Green and The White," p. 334, *The Coca Leaf and Cocaine Papers*)

The story of how coca and cocaine use started in Europe and North America is related in many ways to its traditional use by the South American Indians. Most early commercial products were made from the whole coca leaf. In Europe, Angelo Mariani produced a coca wine which gained wide popular acceptance. John Styth Pemberton, a pharmacist in Georgia, developed in 1886 a tonic soda water as a temperance drink (non-alcoholic) which he called Coca-Cola. Both products were sold as elixirs and the positive benefits to good health were their advertised features. A host of similar and even stronger products appeared on the market and the abuse of purified cocaine became a media sensation. Cocaine was removed from Coca-Cola in 1903, and in 1914 cocaine became illegal in the U.S.

Coca is esteemed by the Indians as an aphrodisiac, and is reputed to insure longevity with unimpaired sexual powers. Nineteenth century observers commented on the incredible longevity of some Ecuadorean Indians, with life spans stretching up to 100 years or more.

Eleanor Carroll, NIDA Res. Monograph 13, 1977.

Although coca is native to Peru and Bolivia, it has been successfully cultivated in a variety of climates and countries including Colombia, Jamaica, Ecuador, Brazil, Chile, Java, Ceylon, India, France, and the United States. For further information on the cultivation of coca, see *Mama Coca* by Antonil, published by Hassle Free Press (London), Chapter Six.

Of the various species of *coca,* only two have been used as primary sources of cocaine, and it is these upon which we will focus. *Erythroxylum coca,* called Huanaco, is primarily cultivated on the eastern slopes of the Andes in Bolivia and Peru. Its greenish-colored leaves are elliptically shaped with parallel longitudinal lines on the underside of the leaf. It has a haylike odor. The plant grows well in altitudes between 500–1500 meters where the climate is favorably tropical, high in rainfall, moderate in temperature, and the soils are mineral rich and well drained. *E. coca* is the most important commercial species of coca and is used to make the majority of the world's cocaine. In Peru, the leaves from *E. coca* represent 95% of the total annual crop. As with the other varieties of coca, the alkaloid content is variable both in amount and composition, depending on where it is grown. A variety of *E. coca* called *Ipadu* or *Amazonian coca* is cultivated in the western Amazon of Brazil, Colombia, and Peru. This variety is propagated by cuttings rather than seeds, and prefers moderate temperatures and well-drained soils. The plant itself is taller and

(Continued on page 29)

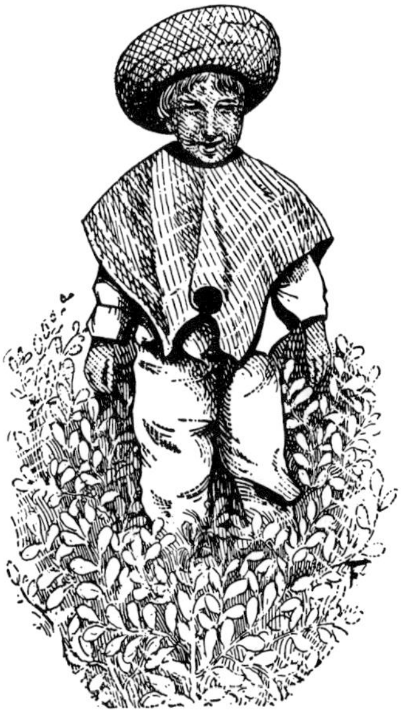

A Little Coca Picker (by Brettes, from *History of Coca,* W.G. Mortimer)

Advertisement for Vin Mariani, Paris, c. 1890. Angelo Mariani marketed this stimulating coca-leaf wine, predecessor to coca-based soft drinks, for physicians and fashionable connoisseurs alike. Its exact recipe was a closely guarded secret, but Mariani received and published twelve volumes of testimonials to its tonic virtues from many notables, including Jules Verne, Sarah Bernhardt, the Czar and Czarina of Russia, Thomas Edison, and Queen Victoria. Pope Leo XIII awarded Mariani a Gold Medal for this elixir made from the Divine Plant of the Incas.

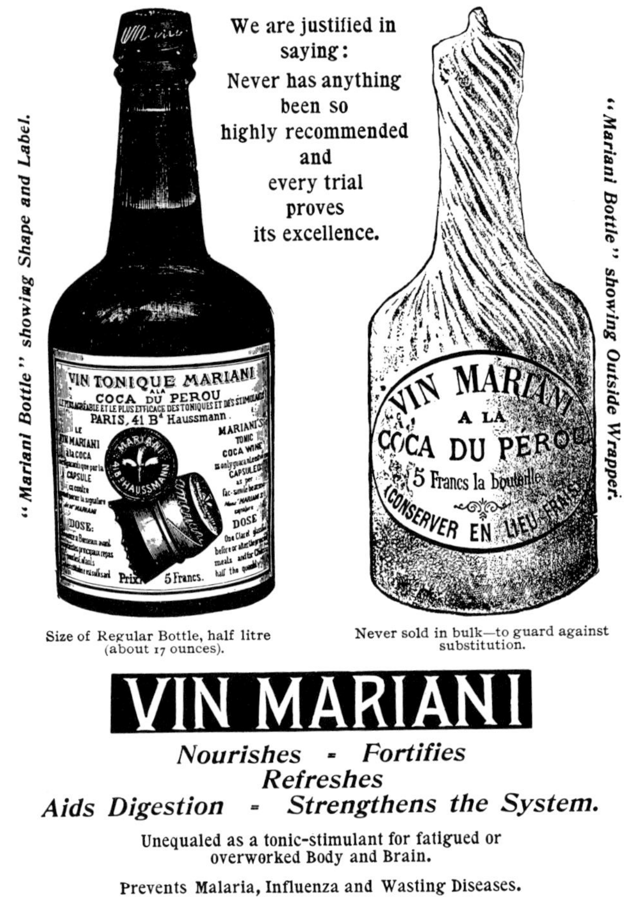

TESTIMONIAL QUOTES FROM THE MARIANI ALBUM 1884–1913

Thomas Alva Edison.

"Monsieur Mariani, I take pleasure in sending you one of my photographs for publication in your Album. Yours very truly."

Camille Flammarion (an astronomer who founded the French Society of Astronomers).

"Solar rays in bottles."

Charles Gounod (composer of symphonies and operas).
"To my good friend Mariani, beneficial revealer of this admirable coca wine from Peru, which has so often restored my strength."

Cardinal Lavigerie.
"Your coca from America gave my European priests the strength to civilise Asia and Africa."

Pope Leo XIII sent a gold medal to Mariani through a Cardinal with the following letter:
"Rome, January 2, 1898. His Holiness has deigned to commission me to thank the distinguished donor in His holy name, and to demonstrate His gratitude in a material way as well. His Holiness does me the honour of presenting Mr. Mariani with a gold medal containing His venerable coat-of-arms."

William McKinley (President of the United States).
"Executive Mansion, Washington, June 14, 1898. My dear Sir, Please accept thanks on the President's behalf and on my own for your courtesy in sending a case of the celebrated Vin Mariani, with whose tonic virtues I am already acquainted, and will be happy to avail myself of in the future as occasion may require. Very truly yours, John Addison Porter, Secretary to the President."

Auguste Rodin.
"To Mariani, who spreads coca. Your friend."

Jules Verne.
"Since a single bottle of Mariani's extraordinary coca wine guarantees a lifetime of a hundred years, I shall be obliged to live until the year 2700! Well, I have no objections! Yours very gratefully."

ESSENTIALS FOR CULTIVATION OF COCA

The temperature in which Coca is grown must be equable, of about 18° C. (64.4° F.). If the mean exceeds 20° C. (68° F.), the plant loses strength and the leaf assumes a dryness which always indicates that it is grown in too warm a situation, and though the leaves may be more prolific, they have not the delicate aroma of choice Coca.

* * *

A peculiar earth is required for the most favorable cultivation of Coca, one rich in mineral matter, yet free from limestone, which is so detrimental that even when it is in the substratum of a vegetable soil the shrub grown over it will be stunted and the foliage scanty. While the young Coca plants may thrive best in a light, porous soil, such as that in the warmer valleys, the full grown shrub yields a better quality of leaf when grown in clay.

* * *

This, commonly mixed with organic matter and salts from the decaying vegetation, or that of the trees burned to make a clearing, affords what might be termed a virgin earth—*terra franche ou normale*—which requires no addition of manures for invigoration. In the conservatory it has been found, after careful experimentation, that a mixture of leaf mould and sand—*terre de bruyère,* forms the best artificial soil for the Coca plant.

Aside from an appropriate soil that is well drained, there is another important element to the best growth of Coca, and that is a humid atmosphere. Indeed, in the heart of the montaña it is either hazy or drizzling during some portion of the day throughout the year, the intense glare of the tropical sun being usually masked by banks of fog, so that it would seem that one living here is dwelling in the clouds.

Mortimer, *History of Coca.*

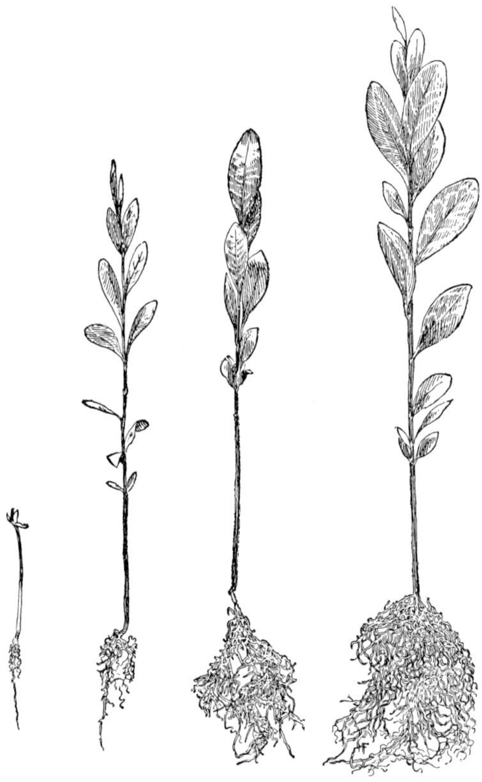

Young coca plants, showing fibrous root. —*Conservatory of Mariani.* (from Mortimer, *History of Coca.*)

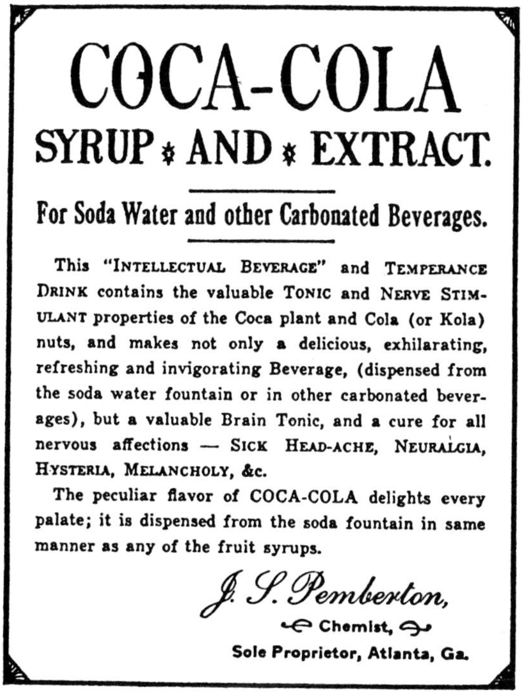

Advertisement for spring 1887. 1,049 gallons were sold that year. (John Graff, *High Times*, 1977.)

Few recall to what extraordinary degree Americans were attached to cocaine around the turn of the century. Coca-Cola, of course, was originally indebted to the cocaine base of its syrup for the pause that refreshed. But it was just one of a host of elixirs, tonics, patent medicines and just plain soda pop available over the counter and through the mail that carried a powerful coke kick. Koa-Kola, Kola-Ade, Koca-Nola, Cafe-Coca Compound, Celery Cola, Coke Extract, Dr. Don's Kola, Vani-Kola Compound Syrup, Rococola, Wiseola—all were beverages containing cocaine that were commonly available at the grocery store.

Jerry Carroll, *New West*, 1980.

(Continued from page 25)

more spindly than Huanaco and has weak branches and relatively large elliptical leaves which are blunt or rounded at the apex. Its underside lacks the characteristic parallel lines. Amazonian coca contains very little true cocaine and is primarily used for chewing by the people who cultivate it.

Erythroxylum novogranatense is native to Colombia, Venezuela, and parts of Central America. In Colombia, it grows in the Sierra Nevada de Santa Marta and in the rugged mountains of Cauca and Hucha. This species is highly resistant to drought and prefers a hot, dry habitat. It is a bushier plant than *E. coca,* with smaller, narrower, and thinner leaves which are bright yellowish green in color and rounded at the apex. Its leaves contain large amounts of methyl salicylate which give it a wintergreen odor. However, its true cocaine content is much lower than that of *E. coca.* In Colombia, where coca cultivation is

SPECIES OF COCA AND THEIR CHARACTERISTICS

Genus, Species	ERYTHROXYLUM COCA		ERYTHROXYLUM NOVOGRANATENSE	
Varieties	coca	ipadu	novogranatense	truxillense
Origin	montaña region of eastern Andes: Ecuador, Peru, and Bolivia, mainly between 500-1500m	western Amazon of Brazil, Colombia, and Peru	Colombia, Venezuela and Central America, Sierra Nevada de Santa Marta and rugged mountains of Cauca and Hucha	desert coast of Peru and in adjacent arid valley of the Rio Maranon, Truxillo region on the north coast of Peru
Description of plant and/or leaves	pointed leaves, parallel longitudinal lines on leaf undersides	tall, spindly shrub with long weak branches and relatively large elliptical leaves which are blunt or rounded at the apex; flowers have a shorter flusher pedicel and a markedly denticulate staminal tube only short styled morphs	large bush plant with small, narrow, thin, and bright yellow-green leaves which are rounded	up to 3 m tall with multiple trunks reaching 4cm in diameter; branches are dense erect and spread leaves narrowly elliptical to oblong—lanceolate 20-65mm long; medium to light green above pale green to glossy green beneath and midrib fluted with slight medial ridge
Odor	grassy or haylike		wintergreen	wintergreen
Climate	favorable tropical environment with high rainfall, moderate temperatures and well drained mineral rich soils; moist cool	does not like intense heat or poorly drained soils, short-lived	hot, seasonably dry habitat resistant to drought	has been cultivated in arid, desert climate and wet montaña habitat of Colombia; even more tolerant to drought; prefers desert conditions
Adaptability	very little	very little	will survive under a wide range of environmental conditions. Resistant to drought.	
Means of propagation	seeds	cuttings	seeds	seeds
Commercial uses	most important commercial species providing by far the largest supply of coca leaves and cocaine; 95% of Peru's crop	used for chewing	illegal in Colombia; grown illegally for coca chewing and cocaine production	principal variety used in beverage industry owing to its high content of essential oils and flavors—several hundred tons exported to N.Y. for preparation of extracts, used in making Coca-Cola
% Alkaloids	0.5-1.0	unknown	1.0-2.5	1.0-2.5
% Cocaine of total alkaloid content	70-90	very little	20-50	20-50

illegal, illicit crops of *E. novogranatense* are cultivated for local chewing and for illicit cocaine manufacture. While this species has shown great adaptability to other climates, it has also been found that the alkaloid composition and quantity will vary with the climate and soil. An example of this is Java coca, which was adapted from *E. novogranatense*. Until World War II, this variety provided most of the raw materials for the world's supply of pharmaceutical cocaine. While its alkaloid content is even higher in Java than in Colombia, its true cocaine content is much lower.

On the desert coast of Peru and in the adjacent arid valley of the Rio Marañón, a variety of *E. novogranatense* is grown. It has been named *Trujillo* after the region in Peru where it is grown. The leaves of *E. novogranatense* var. truxillense provide only 5% of Peru's annual harvest, and most of this is exported to the United States for use as a flavoring agent in Coca-Cola. The remaining leaves are locally consumed (chewed) by natives who value them for their great aromatic qualities and palatability.

E. novogranatense var. truxillense has been cultivated in both arid and wet climates with great success. Its adaptability and resistance to drought are even greater than Colombian coca, since it actually prefers desert conditions. The plants are propagated by seeds and may grow as tall as 3 meters with multiple trunks reaching 4 centimeters in diameter. The leaves are narrowly elliptic to oblong, 20–65 millimeters long, and 10–25 millimeters wide. The topsides are medium to light green in color and pale green underneath. The midrib is flat with a slight medial ridge.

Chapter Two

The Alkaloids

Very little is known about the physiological activity of the associate alkaloids of the coca plant, and still less about their effects in combination. The necessity of looking into the possible importance of these other compounds is emphasized by the fact that an Indian will frequently reject the bitter coca leaves with the highest percentage of cocaine in favor of the sweeter leaves which are richer in the more aromatic alkaloids.

Richard T. Martin,
Economic Botany, 1970.

Cocaine is only one of the alkaloids contained in the leaves of the plant *Erythroxylum coca*. Varying amounts of several other similar alkaloids will also be present, depending on the particular species of coca which is used, where it is grown, and the manner by which it is refined.

Most uncut illicit cocaine will consist primarily of three or four alkaloids; these include: *cocaine, cocamine* (truxillines), *cinnamylcocaine*, and the *hygrines*. In addition, *benzoylecgonine* is found in minute quantities or in larger amounts when the cocaine has decomposed. *Tropacocaine* is rarely present in South American coca but does occur significantly in Java coca.

As well as the alkaloids which naturally occur in coca, mixed alkaloid cocaine will often containe *ecgonine*. As with benzoylecgonine, ecgonine is produced when the cocaine has decomposed. This can happen intentionally, but is usually caused by attempting to force a higher yield from the leaves, paste, or base.

Licit pharmaceutical cocaine, used in medicine as a local anesthetic, is manufactured legally under optimum laboratory conditions. In this process all alkaloids which can be converted to cocaine are used. This includes three alkaloids which have ecgonine at the core of their molecule: cocaine (methyl benzoylecgonine), cinnamylcocaine (methyl cinnamylecgonine), and cocamine (methyl truxilloylecgonine). The molecules are split into their main parts, the ecgonine portion saved, and the rest eliminated. Once isolated, the ecgonine may be synthetically converted to cocaine (methyl benzoylecgonine).

The advantage of this process is a higher yield of cocaine from coca which contains predominately cocamine or cinnamylcocaine. The disadvantage of the process is that it is technically demanding and requires exacting technique, special chemicals, and sophisticated laboratory equipment.

The ecgonine conversion process has been used by chemists since 1885 but is virtually unknown to the "cooks" of South America who make most of the illicit cocaine. Prior to its discovery, cocaine was refined in much the same way that is used by illicit manufacturers today. While both techniques begin with the extraction of all alkaloids, the illicit process (when properly conducted) seeks to eliminate all alkaloids but cocaine. The pharmaceutical process eliminates only those alkaloids which cannot be made into cocaine.

It should be pointed out that only the ecgonine process will totally eliminate the related alkaloids so that the only alkaloid at the end is cocaine. The illicit process will always leave traces of the other alkaloids. Whereas pharmaceutical cocaine hydrochloride will be 89.27% cocaine base by weight, illicit mixed-alkaloid cocaine hydrochloride will rarely be more than 80% cocaine base. When the illicit process is used on species of coca which have high concentrations of other alkaloids, the amount of cocaine base may drop to 50% or lower.

When discussing the illicit process, it is important to consider the conditions under which it is performed. The illicit processor rarely has access to the wide range of quality chemicals available in the United States and Europe. The process is carried out by "cooks" who know little about chemistry and routinely use substitute solvents

Chemical Structure of Cocaine

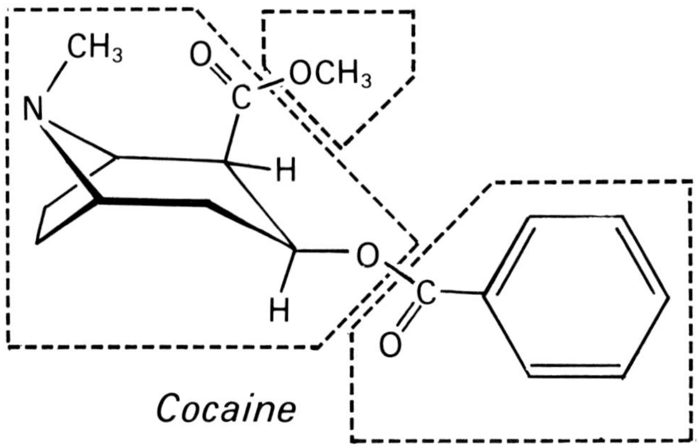

The cocaine molecule is made up of three building blocks. If chemical conditions become too acidic or too basic the cocaine molecule readily breaks down into these three pieces.

Decomposition of Cocaine

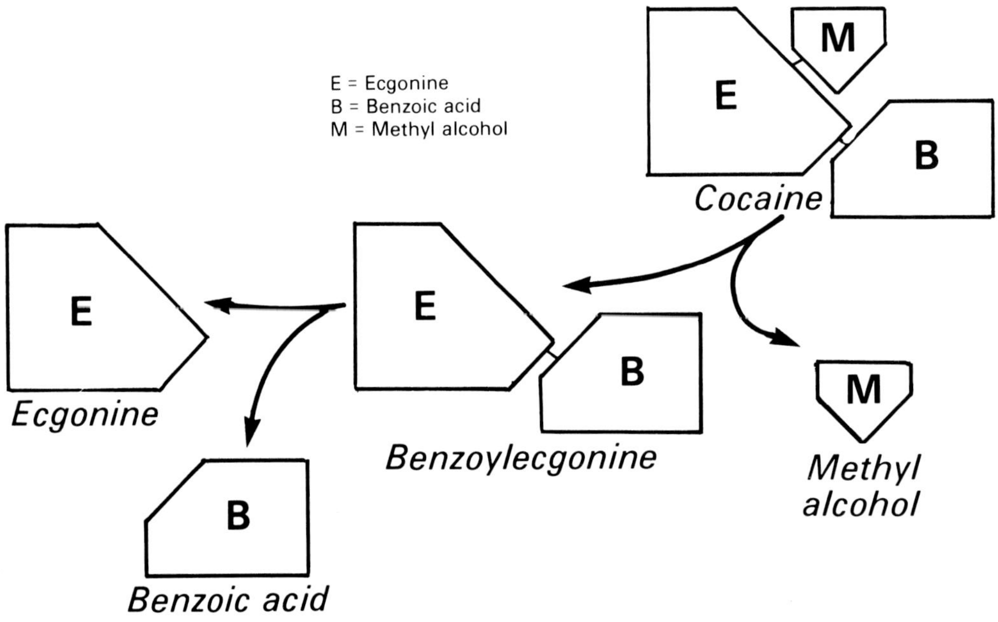

and chemicals, depending on what is available. (This would be impossible when using the pharmaceutical process).

As a South American "cook" once said, "All you need to make cocaine is three buckets and two sheets." Many cooks actually use this method. The work is done in make-shift laboratories more reminiscent of kitchens, and the sheets (complete with multiple kilos) are often hung on a clothesline to dry in the sun. Time is of the essence, and one never knows when a cocaine kitchen may have to be moved at a moment's notice. Lengthy procedures are abbreviated to meet this criterion and quality is often sacrificed in the process.

When the Colombian cook saw the sophisticated lab he said "all you need to make cocaine is three buckets and two sheets." Once in the remote mountains of Central America we ran out of filter paper while preparing to crystalize a batch. We went into town, rented a hotel room, stole the sheets and headed back to the hills where we finished the job.

Colombian Cook

There are three kinds of laboratories which deal with different parts of the procedure. The *pasta lab* is usually located at or near the growing area and is used to extract all the alkaloids in the form of a water-soluble paste. This crude cocaine sulfate, called pasta, is far less bulky than the leaves themselves, and the extraction procedure and laboratory requirements are simple enough to be performed by the coca growers. (It takes 100–150 kilos of dry leaves to produce one kilo of dry pasta.) All that is required is to soak the dried leaves in water, add a strong alkali like lime to release the alkaloids, and stir in a solvent like kerosene or gasoline which will dissolve the alkaloids while remaining separate from the water. The water is drained out the bottom of the container and the gasoline is poured out the top. Once the gasoline has been separated, sulfuric acid is added to precipitate the alkaloids. The precipitate, called pasta, is separated from the gasoline by filtration and put out in the sun to dry. (In Bolivia, where the predominant alkaloid is cocaine, hydrochloric acid is often substituted for sulfuric acid, and the resultant hydrochloride is the finished product.)

The dry pasta is usually tannish brown, the color coming from plant material, dirt, etc. It usually contains all compounds which will precipitate with lime and dissolve in gasoline. If a stronger alkali is used, more compounds will be present.

The next step of the process is to convert the pasta to base. This is usually done in a *base lab* located in Colombia and is a very critical part of the procedure since it determines the amount and proportions of different alkaloids which will be present in the finished product. Parts of this conversion are routinely left out due to the time involved, weight losses, and potential risk to the cocaine. When properly performed, the conversion to base will eliminate cinnamylcocaine and the hygrines, as well as most organic impurities.

A look at the techniques of the "cooks."

"They were crystallizing several kilos and discovered they didn't have a big enough container. I was sent out to get it and came back with a large plastic garbage can. They got to work and I got laid back. Screams drew me to the laboratory where the South American chef had his foot in the can trying to plug the hole that the ether ate through the plastic and his assistant was scooping up the flood off the rug back into the trash can. We had to hold back the owner of the house as we cut up the rug, but the chef managed to recover 90% of the coke."

Manuel the Mule

The conversion is properly performed by dissolving the pasta in water and adding sulfuric acid to further acidify the solution. Potassium permanganate is added to the solution, causing it to turn a violet color. This oxidation process does not appreciably affect the cocaine, but the oils and impurities are attacked almost immediately. The critical part of the process is deciding when to stop the action of the permanganate by adding an alkali. If the decision is made too early, the resultant base will contain more impurities and other alkaloids; if the decision is made too late, some cocaine will be destroyed by the permanganate. There is hardly an experienced cook who has not overoxidized the pasta at one time or another. Never was it more true that "close only counts in horseshoes."

The owners of the pasta are not involved for the fun of it—their purpose is to make money. The loss of a quantity of cocaine due to overoxidation of the pasta is hardly an effective means of increasing the profit, so, more often than not, this part of the process is eliminated. Why take the chance when the cocaine will sell anyway?

Pasta which is converted to base without being oxidized with permanganate rarely results in cocaine hydrochloride which is over 60% cocaine base. Cocaine hydrochloride made from properly oxidized base may be as much as 82% cocaine base.

The last step of the process is to convert the base to "crystal," the South American term for cocaine hydrochloride. This is usually done in a *crystal lab* located in or near a major city in Colombia. The base is dissolved in ether, and hydrochloric acid is added to precipitate the cocaine hydrochloride crystals. These are collected by filtration and are then dried. It is rare for this process to be performed with less than three kilos, and as many as fifty may be done at one time. The crystallization is performed as quickly as possible, taking as little as fifteen minutes where a more professional procedure might take hours.

Since most illicit cocaine is made the quick way, with the emphasis on quantity, it often contains an alkaloid proportion similar to that which existed in the leaves themselves. This is not necessarily bad because most consumers of cocaine seem to prefer the mellower high of mixed-alkaloid cocaine to the speedy but clear high of the pharmaceutical product. One must remember that, in medicine, cocaine is used as a local anesthetic; the presence of other alkaloids makes it less effective as such. However, when the cocaine is used as a recreational drug, the same reasoning may not hold true.

Aside from cocaine, the alkaloids which are of the most interest to the consumer are cocamine and the hygrines. This is of course due to the large amount of these substances which are present in illicit cocaine.

To date, some fourteen alkaloids have been isolated from varieties of the plant. Pharmacologists have burdened us with the notion that drug plants must owe their properties to a single "active principle" that can be isolated, synthesized, studied, and administered in pure form. This notion may be helpful to pharmacologists in making their experiments simpler, but it is disastrous to the rest of us because it leads us away from natural green medicines in the direction of white powders with far higher potentials for abuse.

Andrew Weil,
The Marriage of the Sun and Moon, 1980.

Cocamine* (truxilline) was first discovered in what was then called Trujillo coca and was for many years confused with cocaine due to the remarkable similarities between the two and the difficulty in separating them. Its chemical formula is very close to that of cocaine, the main difference being the kind of acid which is produced when the molecule decomposes. Cocaine decomposes to methyl alcohol, *benzoic acid*, and ecgonine, while cocamine breaks down to methyl alcohol, *truxillic acid,* and ecgonine. This difference results in an alkaloid which is considerably less active than cocaine, with little or no anesthetic value and distinctly different psychoactive qualities. Cocamine acts

* Cocamine (truxilline) is actually a group of five compounds with the same molecular composition but slight differences in geometry (stereoisomers). The chemical behavior is therefore complex because a group of compounds is involved.

PRIMARY COCA ALKALOIDS AND THEIR PROPERTIES

	Description	Melting Point °C	Decomposition Products
Cocaine	colorless crystals or white crystalline powder with no odor and slightly bitter taste	96-98	ecgonine methyl alcohol benzoic acid
Cocamine (Truxillines)	white amorphous powder with dirty odor and very bitter taste	80	ecgonine methyl alcohol truxillic acid
Cinnamylcocaine	colorless needles	121	ecgonine methyl alcohol cinnamic acid
Hygrines	colorless, volatile oil with cat-urine-like odor and very bitter taste	193-5 bp*	hygric acid
Tropacocaine	needles	49	benzoic acid ψ tropine
Benzoylecgonine	colorless crystals, ortho-rhombic prisms or needles	86-92	ecgonine benzoic acid
Ecgonine	crystals, monoclinic prisms	198	

**boiling point*

on the muscular system while cocaine acts on the nervous system. Cocamine is amorphous (noncrystalline), and when present with cocaine will lessen its crystallinity and diminish its brilliance. The taste of cocamine is more bitter than cocaine, with little or no numbing effect. The effects of consuming cocaine which has a significant amount of cocamine will be more physical in nature, lacking the clarity of cocaine. It may actually seem to cause drowsiness.

The hygrines were first thought of as a decomposition product produced during the manufacture of cocaine. They are in fact a natural component of the coca leaf and may be present in quantities as great as 30% of the total alkaloid content. The presence of hygrine in illicit cocaine is often due to the manufacturer's desire to increase the weight of the cocaine. In order for hygrine to precipitate at the same time as cocaine, an excess of hydrochloric acid

I had read in the literature that the smell of dirty sox in cocaine indicated the presence of cocamine and/or hygrine. Imagine my surprise when Cruel Raoul came over and pulled out his stash carefully concealed in his dirty sox. I begged to keep the sox, to no avail.

David Lee

must be used. This often results in partial decomposition of the cocaine molecule. (If the extra acid is not used, most of the hygrine will remain in the solution from which the cocaine has been removed.) The cocaine decomposition is the reason that an overabundance of hygrine is usually accompanied by benzoylecgonine and ecgonine. A sweet smell, reminiscent of wintergreen, is also caused by the breakdown, not by the hygrine.

The hygrines are colorless, volatile oils which are extremely alkaline and possess a very bitter taste. They do not dull the appearance of the cocaine as will cocamine, but they will increase its tendency to attract moisture from the air. Since they possess little or no psychoactive qualities of their own, they will merely lessen the stimulation of cocaine. The excess hydrochloric acid, added when the hygrine was precipitated, is very irritating to the nasal membranes. When the nose neutralizes the excess acid, the hygrine becomes insoluble in water and is poorly absorbed, so it further irritates the nose.

Significant amounts of cocamine and hygrine are found in the leaves of *Erythroxylum novogranatense*. While they may be present in other species of coca, the amount will be minute by comparison. It is therefore logical to assume that mixed-alkaloid cocaine containing large amounts of these alkaloids originated in Colombia or Peru.

Chapter Three

Understanding the Cocaine Trade

Despite repeated half-hearted government attempts to prohibit new planting and to encourage sowing of substitute crops, the ever-growing demand for the raw material of the "champagne of drugs" is spreading coca farming across stony mountain sides, freshly cleared jungle, and even across the thriving coffee and citrus farms of the Bolivian Yungas, steadily being chopped down to make way for the more profitable coca bushes.

Timothy Ross,
LA Times, 1981.

Most cocaine consumers are in agreement that it has become increasingly difficult to obtain high quality illicit cocaine. Prices have risen, quality has dropped, and the alternatives are few. While this is due to a variety of circumstances, the cocaine market, like any other, is governed by the laws of supply and demand. When the demand greatly exceeds the supply, it becomes a sellers' market, a condition which rarely benefits the consumer.

The amount of illicit cocaine which is consumed annually in the United States has increased dramatically in the past 5 years and the demand put on suppliers has risen accordingly. Nowhere is this more widely felt than in South America where the coca leaves which produce the cocaine are grown. The need for larger quantities of leaves from which cocaine can be made has prompted increased coca production throughout South America. Cultivation has extended to remote areas which for various environmental reasons were never considered prime sources of leaves. The result of changes in climate and soil conditions on coca is usually a lowering of the cocaine content and an increased concentration of the related alkaloids. The suppliers are largely unaware of these changes and most don't really care. In the kitchens of Colombia, "If its an alkaloid, its cocaine," and that's that.

It requires 100–150 kilos of dry leaves to produce one kilo of dry, high quality pasta. The extreme difference in volume makes it far more practical for the pasta to be made at or near the growing area. Most often, it is the *farmer* himself who performs this simple process. A small harvest may yield as little as an ounce of pasta. A larger harvest may yield perhaps a pound. Either way, it is hardly enough to satisfy those hungry gringo noses.

Every few months, the ten or twelve farmers who comprise each growing area will be visited by a *guia* (guide). This person is usually of the same nationality as the farmers, and it is his job to obtain the pasta from the entire area and sell it to a *buyer*. The guide will often meet the buyer (usually a Colombian) at the Peruvian/Colombian border and escort him to and from the growing area. The buyer will rarely attempt to go directly to the farmers, whose loyalty is to their own kind. Any such infringement on the guide's "territorial rights" is sufficient ground to eliminate the buyer.

The buyer usually represents one of the larger organizations in Colombia. He obtains the pasta, usually no more than three kilos per trip, and transports it to a *base lab* somewhere in Colombia. Other buyers who represent the same organization will bring their pasta to the same base lab. The pasta is combined with little regard to variances in quality or origin, and is made into base which may then be transported to a crystal lab located in or near one of the major cities in Colombia.

The *crystal lab* receives base from many base labs. The bases are combined (regardless of qualitative differences) and crystallized. This resultant cocaine hydrochloride is not from Colombia, and it's really not from Peru or Bolivia either. Its origin would more accurately be termed Potpourri since it involves the materials and labor of as many as 2000 farmers, 200 guides, 200 buyers, 20 base labs, and several crystal labs — all this before entering the United States.

The majority of illicit cocaine which is smuggled into the U.S.A. comes from Potpourri. It arrives by air or sea in massive loads weighing as much as 300 kilos. In such large shipments there are always variations in quality. The whiter cocaine is considered to be the purest and will go for the highest price. Distributors in the United States are usually required to take a certain number of the discolored kilos in order to obtain some of the "better" product. When scientific testing is used, it is often found that whiter does not necessarily mean better.

"Stick a pin almost anywhere in the South American map and you hit a plantation, or a laboratory, or a grass warehouse or an airstrip," a U.S. State Department narcotics specialist told me with pessimistic hyperbole. "There is probably nothing short of communist revolution or nuclear obliteration that will stop it." . . .

. . . Continent-wide cocaine production now totals more than 100 tons a year, with local consumption and confiscations accounting for less than a quarter. More than two-thirds of exports go to the United States, but European demand is climbing steadily.

Timothy Ross,
LA Times, 1981.

The smuggler usually deals with as few people as possible. He sells or fronts his merchandise to a select number of wholesalers who deal in various parts of the country. They travel to the cocaine's port of entry, usually Florida, to inspect the load and arrange for transportation of the cocaine to their distribution area. Since many kilos are likely to be involved, the load is rarely examined except for its aesthetic properties (look, smell, and taste). The wholesaler knows that there will be variations in quality from bag to bag and he is rarely allowed to choose the kilos he prefers. More often than not, it's all or nothing at all.

Once the cocaine has arrived at a safe house in the wholesaler's territory, it is weighed, inventoried, and perhaps given its first close examination. This may range from a careful analysis of quality to a simple foil burn test. A measure of the product's value is often determined by how many times it can be cut and still be saleable. Up to this point, if the cocaine has been cut, it was usually done without the knowledge of the people in charge. It is often workers within the organization who will attempt to make a little extra by diluting the cocaine with a substance of lesser value. It is therefore not uncommon for a load which has been inspected in Florida to have changed by the time it reaches its destination.

A wholesaler rarely sells less than a kilo at a time, usually more and to several major distributors. The smuggler, wholesalers, and major distributors are the upper echelon of the cocaine business. The volume of product they handle is often too great to permit either grading or

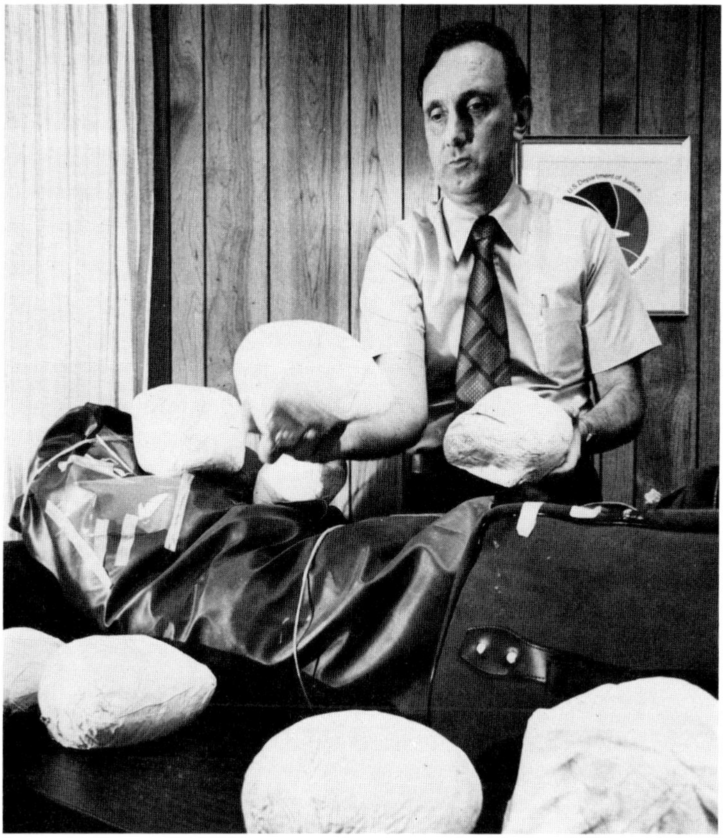

Allan Pringle, drug enforcement officer, holds package of cocaine. *Oakland Tribune* 10/20/80. (Courtesy of Wide World Photos)

adulteration. While kilos may be as different as night and day they are just more products to sell and are all handled in the same way; poured from bag to bag like sacks of flour with little regard about spilling or exact weights.

From the major distributors on, cocaine dealers are hard to characterize since they come from all walks of life. Most use it themselves but deal primarily to make money in addition to earning what they use. In general, the smaller the volume a quantity dealer handles, the further down the line he is and the more likely his product has been adulterated.

To the gram buyer of cocaine, it is his connection who is the source. While quite detached from the politics of the larger cocaine trade, his customers still depend on him for information regarding the nature and purity of the cocaine. Often, the source is as uninformed as the customer, and since he is likely to have a financial interest in the sale,

"We have someone jump on $500,000 bond almost every week. When somebody can put up $500,000 or $1 million bond straight cash, that's a clue anybody can see: We're never going to see that guy again.

Assistant U.S. Attorney Pat Sullivan—after a suspect of a $9 million (874 pounds of cocaine base) arrest had posted bond of $1 million in cash. The suspect did not appear for trial. AP Miami 1980.

he may be the least interested in passing along meaningful information about the cocaine. An unscrupulous source may find that he can increase his profits by adulterating or lightweighting the cocaine. The consumer who has no alternative may find each purchase to be an expensive lesson.

Can anything be done to end this sorry cycle of bad cocaine, bad bargains and bad karma? Legalization would do it, but that step is hardly imminent. A consumer boycott, a refusal to buy adulterated crap, would stop it too. Not that this is a likely prospect either, but it would work. Dealers, after all, are merchants, and if their customers won't buy inferior goods, they'll soon make sure that something better is available.

Richard Ashley, *High Times,* 1979.

The type of source which is most often encountered by the gram buyer of cocaine is the dealer-user. This person defrays the cost of consuming cocaine by selling moderate quantities. Contrary to the media image of a cocaine dealer, the dealer-user is usually far from being a "superfly." In many cases he may be a marijuana dealer who occasionally sells cocaine. This person normally makes money selling marijuana, but tends to take cocaine as his profit on cocaine transactions. The successful dealer-user must usually make a quick turnover in order to avoid consuming more than just the profit. Where this is not possible, the cocaine is often adulterated so as to avoid a loss.

The most common purchase made by the dealer-user is one-quarter of one ounce, 7 grams. This is broken down into grams and half-grams which are usually packaged in a hand-folded envelope called a bindle. The selling price is variable and is rarely concurrent with quality, but the typical dealer-user will try to make one to 2 grams on the purchase of a quarter-ounce. If the cost of the 7 grams is 600 dollars, and the dealer-user wants to make 2 grams, he must sell the 5 remaining grams for the 600 dollars he paid for the quarter-ounce. The result is a gram price of 120 dollars. Often, grams are lightweighted in order to increase the profit. The "nine-tenths of a gram per gram" is very common. Applied to the sale of 5 grams, the result is an extra one-half gram to snort or sell. The best way for the gram buyer to avoid being cheated is to understand precisely what he is buying. "Don't be afraid to ask!" is sound consumer advice.

The consumer should understand that constant ingestion of cocaine can impair the user's judgment. When this is combined with poor integrity, the result is often overly adulterated cocaine. A dealer in this condition is more likely to make a questionable purchase in order to maintain his own supply. The cocaine may sell slowly, forcing the

COCAINE TRADE HIERARCHY FROM FARM TO CONSUMER

(THE HISTORY OF A HYPOTHETICAL 300-KILO SHIPMENT)

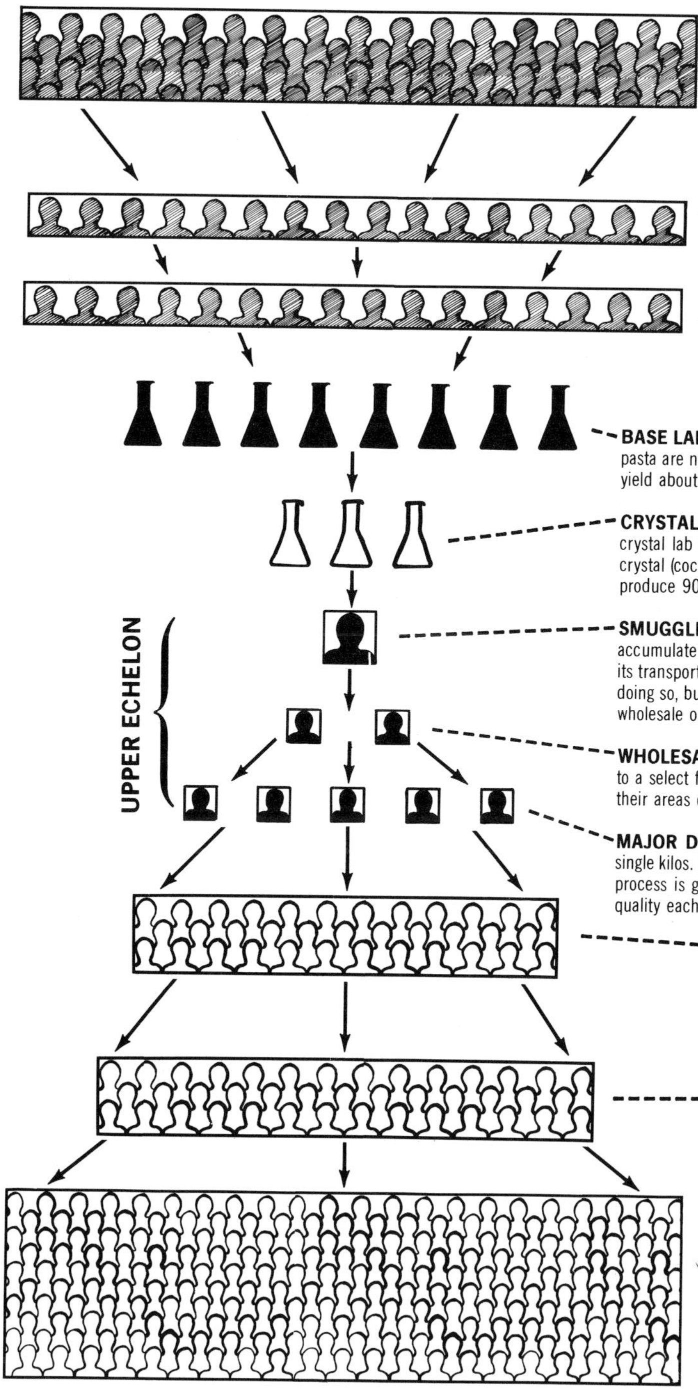

FARMERS: Cultivate coca, harvest & dry leaves, and make the pasta. Every few months, as many as 2000 farmers (working separately) will use a total of 45,000 kilos of dried leaves to make approx. 375 kilos of pasta—which will eventually become the hypothetical 300-kilo shipment. One average farmer's yield of pasta would be less than 200 grams.

GUIDES: Each native guide buys pasta from 10-12 farmers of his own nationality and sells to one (usually) Colombian buyer representing a large organization. He also often escorts the buyer to and from the growing area as his presence there without a guide would not be tolerated by the locals.

BUYERS: Buy pasta from their guides and transport it to their organization's base lab located somewhere in the Colombian countryside.

BASE LABS: Convert pasta to cocaine base. Approx. 1.25 kilos of pasta are needed to make one kilo of base, so 375 kilos of pasta will yield about 300 kilos of base.

CRYSTAL LABS: Base from each of 3-5 base labs is received by a crystal lab in or near a major Colombian city and is converted to crystal (cocaine hydrochloride). One kilo, or 1000 grams, of base will produce 900-1100 grams of cocaine.

SMUGGLER: It will take the yields of several crystal labs to accumulate the 300 kilos of one smuggler's shipment. He will arrange its transportation to the U.S., contacting as few people as possible in doing so, but usually working in collusion with the person managing wholesale operations here.

WHOLESALER: Usually sells multiple-kilo lots at the point of entry to a select few major distributors who transport their purchases to their areas of business.

MAJOR DISTRIBUTORS: Usually buy multiple kilos and sell single kilos. It is at this level that cuts begin to be introduced, and the process is generally repeated at every level, resulting in declining quality each time.

DEALERS: At this stage, an indeterminate series of transactions can take place in which each purchase is smaller: single kilos to pounds, to quarter-pounds, to ounces (with possible adulterations at each step), ending eventually with a purchase by the dealer/user.

DEALER/USER: Buys an ounce or less at a time. Sells to possibly 4-8 consumers (or other dealer/users) in grams and half- or quarter-grams to cover the costs of his own consumption.

CONSUMER: The consumer usually buys one gram or less for personal use. By this point, the 300-kilo shipment has been adulterated so heavily that it consists of 2,500,000 grams which contain only 12% cocaine, and cost at least $100 each for a total of $250,000,000—OR NEARLY $1000 PER GRAM OF ACTUAL COCAINE!

dealer to adulterate the product in order to lower the selling price or to make up for what has been consumed.

If the consumer finds that he is dissatisfied with his source, a determination should be made as to whether the source lacks integrity or expertise. A copy of this book should correct a lack of expertise. A lack of integrity can only be corrected by finding another source for cocaine.

On a more positive note, the dealer who has consistently treated his customers with respect and consideration by supplying a good product at fair weights exhibits good integrity. When such integrity is displayed regularly, the consumer is more likely to be treated consistently in this fashion. However, the nature of the cocaine trade dictates a consumer policy of occasionally double-checking the source. If there is a discrepancy, the buyer should feel free to inform the seller and discuss the transaction. The seller will almost always attempt to satisfy a regular customer who approaches him in a reasonable manner.

Perhaps one of the most important of the unwritten laws of the cocaine trade concerns Cocaine Karma. Success in the cocaine business is often dependent on how a seller treats his customers. A person who misrepresents a product is likely to be caught at his own game. While adulteration or lightweighting may bring more immediate rewards, the long-term effects are apt to be more negative. On the other hand, honest dealers tend to attract honest customers. They may make less money per transaction, but they tend to be around a lot longer.

Chapter Four

The High Cost of Getting High

Give cocaine to a man already wise, schooled to the world, morally forceful, a man of intelligence and self-control. If he be really master of himself, it will do him no harm. He will know it for a snare; he will beware of repeating such experiments as he may make; and the glimpse of his goal may possibly even spur him to its attainment by those means which God has appointed for His saints. But give it to the clod, to the self-indulgent, to the blasé — to the average man, in a word — and he is lost. He says, and his logic is perfect: This is what I want. He knows not, neither can he know, the true path; and the false path is the only one for him. There is cocaine at his need, and he takes it again and again. The contrast between his grub life and his butterfly life is too bitter for his unphilosophic soul to bear; he refuses to take the brimstone with the treacle.

Aleister Crowley,
Cocaine, 1918.

There is little need to enumerate the attractive aspects of cocaine. The increased use of cocaine by people from every walk of life provides ample evidence of the existence of its positive qualities. In fact, the positive aspects are so distinctive that the negative aspects are often unrecognized, misunderstood, or ignored. Nonetheless negative aspects do exist, and an understanding of their nature and a practical knowledge of how to compensate for them should be foremost in the minds of all cocaine users. Since cocaine use over both short and extended periods can lead to many health problems, this will be discussed next.

Cocaine and Health

Cocaine is a stimulant of the central nervous system. It is legally classified as a Schedule II drug with an accepted medical use (as a topical anesthetic) and a high potential for abuse resulting in psychological dependence. The behavioral effects of cocaine vary with purity, dosage, and the way it is taken. The route of intake is *very* critical regarding time, e.g., shooting or base smoking vs. snorting or taking a pill. When "snorted" the initial effects are felt almost immediately with the full effects taking about 15 minutes to develop. The heart rate increases as does body temperature, respiratory rate, and blood pressure. Mental alertness increases and the appetite is depressed. A feeling of physical and mental well-being predominates.

In its pharmacologic action, cocaine, perhaps more than any other of the recognized psychoactive drugs, reinforces and boosts what we recognize as the highest aspirations of American initiative, energy, frenetic achievement, and ebullient optimism (even in the face of great odds). On the coin's darker side of course are exhaustion, paranoia, and violence.

G. R. Gay and D. S. Inaba (in Mulé, 1976).

Depending on the individual, these effects may last for as little as 20 minutes or as long as 2 hours. As the stimulative effects wear off, depression may set in. Blood pressure and heart rate drop to a lower rate than that which existed prior to ingestion. The stronger the initial stimulation, the more pronounced will be the "crash." In fact, the contrast is so great that the user is often inclined to counteract it by ingesting more cocaine.

Prolonged use of cocaine can lead to many health problems. Physically, the chronic user may experience hyperstimulation, headaches, nausea, irregular respiration, anxiety, and possibly convulsions. Over an extended period of time, cocaine use can lead to infections, digestive disorders, severe weight loss, malnutrition, and chronic insomnia. The user may also be faced with many psychological problems, including paranoid delusions, hallucinations, anxiety, depression, and confusion in the decision-making process. Concentration, comprehension, and reaction ability may all be markedly impaired.

While cocaine is not physically addicting, it is very habit forming. The term psychogenetic dependence is often used to describe this condition. Although there is no physical dependence resulting in violent physical reaction to withdrawal, the user thinks he has a physical need for the drug. The difference is a very fine line; if the consumer carried the habit to extremes, the distinction between a real and imagined addiction may not be too relevant. Cocaine certainly affects judgment as to what is real or imagined, and all consumers should keep this in mind.

Periodic abstinence is by far the best means of counteracting these effects. In the absence of abstinence, other measures must be taken. A balanced diet is extremely important, and although the user may not feel like eating,

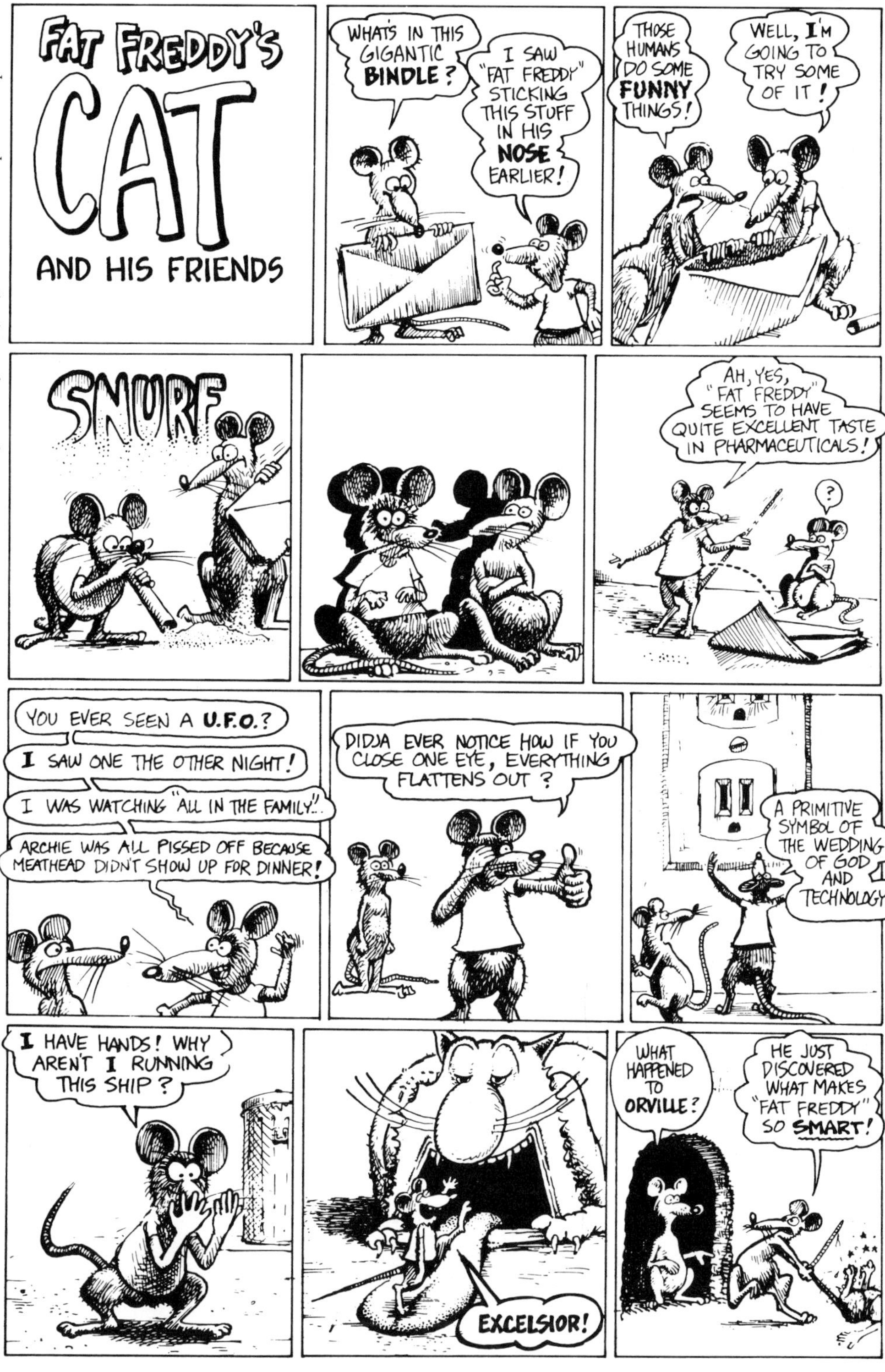
FAT FREDDY'S CAT
AND HIS FRIENDS
WHAT'S IN THIS GIGANTIC BINDLE?
I SAW "FAT FREDDY" STICKING THIS STUFF IN HIS NOSE EARLIER!
THOSE HUMANS DO SOME FUNNY THINGS!
WELL, I'M GOING TO TRY SOME OF IT!
SNURF
AH, YES, "FAT FREDDY" SEEMS TO HAVE QUITE EXCELLENT TASTE IN PHARMACEUTICALS!
?
YOU EVER SEEN A U.F.O.?
I SAW ONE THE OTHER NIGHT!
I WAS WATCHING "ALL IN THE FAMILY."
ARCHIE WAS ALL PISSED OFF BECAUSE MEATHEAD DIDN'T SHOW UP FOR DINNER!
DIDJA EVER NOTICE HOW IF YOU CLOSE ONE EYE, EVERYTHING FLATTENS OUT?
A PRIMITIVE SYMBOL OF THE WEDDING OF GOD AND TECHNOLOGY!
I HAVE HANDS! WHY AREN'T I RUNNING THIS SHIP?
EXCELSIOR!
WHAT HAPPENED TO ORVILLE?
HE JUST DISCOVERED WHAT MAKES "FAT FREDDY" SO SMART!

From the *Adventures of Fat Freddy's Cat*, (1977), Gilbert Shelton. Reprinted with permission.

he must force himself to eat. The first bite is the hardest. Cocaine use burns up energy at an extremely rapid rate, and energy levels must be maintained. Liquid intake is very important since cocaine use dehydrates the body. Taking vitamins, especially B, C and E, will help to counteract cocaine's tendency to deplete them. Cocaine is a stress-producing drug, and even occasional users find that high bodily levels of vitamin B complex help cope with this stress.

Cocaine addiction differs from opiate addiction, and from alcohol and barbiturate addiction, in at least two respects. A cocaine user, even after prolonged use of large doses, does not, if deprived of his drug, suffer from a dramatic withdrawal crisis like alcoholic delirium tremens or like the opiate withdrawal syndrome. The *physical* effects of cocaine withdrawal are minor. This has led many authorities, mistakenly, to classify cocaine as a nonaddicting drug. However, cocaine withdrawal is characterized by a profound psychological manifestation—*depression*—for which cocaine itself appears to the user to be the only remedy; cocaine addiction in this respect resembles tobacco addiction more closely than it resembles opiate addiction or alcoholism. The compulsion to resume cocaine is very strong.

E.M. Brecher, *Licit and Illicit Drugs*, 1972.

Many people find the need to balance the cocaine stimulation with some kind of depressant. Often, this depressant will be alcohol. This can be dangerous if alcohol intake is substituted for water intake. If the body is dehydrated, alcohol is more easily and rapidly absorbed into the bloodstream. In excess, this can result in alcohol poisoning. If the consumer insists on drinking alcohol, drinking extra liquids (water) can lessen the toxic effect of the alcohol.

Cocaine overdoses have been known to occur on amounts of as little as 0.20 gram.

The most common method of ingesting cocaine is by inhalation. This is accomplished by chopping or screening the cocaine into a fine powder and sniffing it into the nasal passages through a straw or from a very small spoon. "Snorting" is a very efficient means of introducing cocaine into the bloodstream because the inner nose membranes are lined with tiny blood vessels. Cocaine entering the nose will settle on the sticky walls of the mucous membranes where it will dissolve almost immediately. It can then be absorbed through the capillary walls, into the bloodstream and on to the brain.

The cocaine totally numbs the area, and the nasal membranes shrink as their blood supply diminishes. Since cocaine constricts the flow of blood in the vein (vasoconstrictor), the mucous membranes will demand the blood which has been withheld as soon as the drug wears off. The nose soon becomes congested, and sneezing and head cold symptoms are likely to follow. Any cocaine which remains undissolved in the nose can cause burns and sores

TREATMENT INTERVENTION FOR COCAINE REACTIONS, A SUMMARY

(This chart was originally published as a guide for health-care professionals in dealing with cocaine overdose.)

Phase	Central Nervous System	Circulatory System	Respiratory System
Early stimulation	Excitement; apprehension; other symptoms of emotional instability Sudden headache Nausea, vomiting "Twitchings" of small muscles, particularly of face, fingers	Pulse varies; probably will slow (Usual) elevation in blood pressure Fall in blood pressure may occur Pallor of skin	Increased respiratory rate *and* depth
Advanced stimulation	Convulsions (tonic and clonic)—resembles grand mal seizure	Increase in both pulse rate *and* blood pressure	Cyanosis, dyspnea, rapid (gasping or irregular) respiration
Depression	Paralysis of muscles Loss of reflexes Unconsciousness Loss of vital functions Death	Circulatory failure No palpable pulse Death	Respiratory failure Ashen-gray cyanosis Death

TREATMENT OF THE "CAINE" REACTION

1. Administration of oxygen; by positive pressure and artificial respiration if necessary.
2. Trendelenburg position (head down). Wrap arms and legs if necessary to increase central return of blood.
3. Inject small amounts of short-acting barbiturates (e.g., 25-50 mg sodium pentothal) if convulsions are present. May be repeated, but gently. Do not force general depressant effect to point of no return. [Note: diazepam (Valium) is more commonly used today.]
4. Administer intravenous stimulants for cardiotonic effect (e.g., phenylephrine 10-20 mg).
5. Keep patient cool, and keep crowds away.
6. General muscle relaxants may be given (e.g., curare, succinylcholine) to facilitate administration of positive-pressure oxygen.
7. Continuously monitor vital signs.

Other than purely supportive respiratory measures, resuscitation efforts should be carried out only in controlled situations (ambulance, hospital) and by experts.

Gay, Sheppard, and Inaba; *International Journal of Addiction* 8(6), 1027-42, 1973.

"Prolonged use of cocaine gives the nose a diffused augmentation of volume and a dull bluish paleness, as if made of gelatin or putty. At the tip of the nose there is freqently a rounded dividing line, and the wings of the nose are slightly swollen. The slang expression used by sniffers to describe the shape of such a nose compares it to the shape of the buttocks. Sniffers recognize each other easily in this way, and cocaine dealers spot prospective clients. The wings of the nose, which are slightly turned up, are constantly in movement. The nostrils are dilated and surrounded by a pink border about one millimeter wide, which gives the impression of a constantly blocked nose, 'astonished nose,' 'plugged nose.' "

Bonvicini, quoted by Leon Natanson (1936). *Coca Leaf and Cocaine Papers*, 1975.

which can eventually lead to degeneration of the membrane or eat through the cartilage itself. This may be prevented by periodically cleaning the nose with some type of nasal douche. Several home recipes for douching are popular, but none are more effective than that used by Michael Aldrich. (See "Tips on Health Care.") The more efficient the cleaning, the less the chance of nasal damage.

The smoking of freebase cocaine is a relatively new phenomenon in the United States which has been rising in popularity at an alarming rate. "Freebase" is the alkaline form of cocaine, the alkaloid itself. When an alkali like ammonium hydroxide is added to a water solution of cocaine hydrochloride, the cocaine (base) is freed from the HCl molecule. It may then be separated from the water by filtration or extraction with a solvent like petroleum ether.* Most freebasers choose the extraction method because it greatly decreases the drying time while allowing the user to create beautiful formations of crystals. With cocaine aesthetics on the decline, this becomes a process which can bring back some visual aesthetics, increasing its appeal.

Freebase is usually consumed in a water pipe which has been specifically designed for the smoking of oils. The bowl of the pipe is designed to accommodate multiple levels of stainless steel screens. The base is placed on the top screen, melted to an oil, and then heated slowly while air is drawn through the stem and into the mouth. Sometimes a rum-soaked (151 proof) burning cotton ball is used for heating the base. The water pipes have the smoke pass through water prior to entering the stem. This cools and smooths out the smoke while acting as a kind of filter for impurities. Often, the base is not heated directly. The glass bowl is heated from the side with a gas torch in order to minimize match or lighter fume inhalation. This also helps

(Continued on page 56)

* A less pure base is sometimes made by dissolving the cocaine hydrochloride in water, making the solution alkaline (sodium bicarbonate is the alkali most often used), and heating the mixture until all the water has evaporated. The waxy base which is produced contains the added alkali and the same adulterants and impurities as did the original cocaine.

DAMAGE TO THE NOSE MUST BE MENDED SURGICALLY

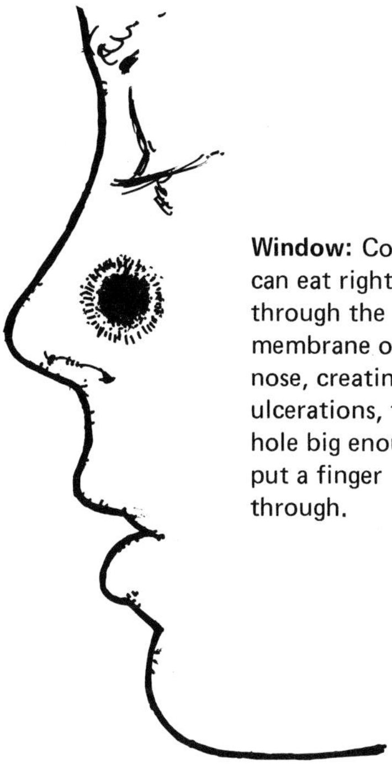

Window: Cocaine can eat right through the septal membrane of the nose, creating first ulcerations, then a hole big enough to put a finger through.

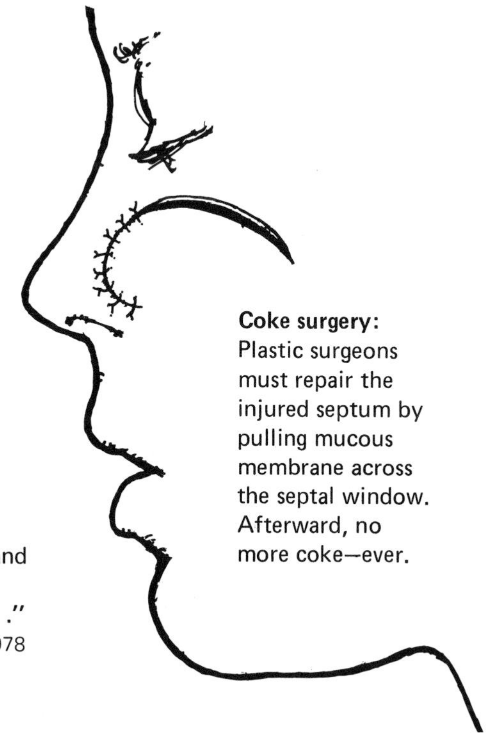

Coke surgery: Plastic surgeons must repair the injured septum by pulling mucous membrane across the septal window. Afterward, no more coke—ever.

"... she was young, she was beautiful, and she had a dime-sized hole between her nostrils from endless cocaine snorting..."

Henry Post, New York Magazine, 1978

TIPS ON HEALTH CARE

Cocaine connoisseurs crush, chop, or screen the coke to a fine powder, and use small doses—aiming it high up inside the nasal cavity.

Beyond that, health care consists of three simple rules. First, don't neglect eating, even if you're not hungry. This also means keeping your levels of bodily fluids up to par by drinking plenty of water or fruit juices (not alcohol). Cocaine—especially if you're also smoking marijuana—dries up the membranes on which it is placed, and also dries up bodily fluids generally. Without adequate food and fluids, your body cannot function normally. The exhaustion that most users feel after a cocaine run is the signal that you should let that wonderful machine—your body—recuperate with the basics of sleep, food, and water.

Secondly, take your vitamins. The extra stress that cocaine causes in your energy and life-support systems quickly depletes your vitamin levels. The coca plant itself offers a clue to the vitamins and minerals appropriate for use with cocaine. One hundred grams of *Erythroxylum coca* provides more than the daily Recommended Dietary Allowance of vitamins A, B_2, and E, calcium, iron, and phosphorus, as well as a healthy complement of vitamin C, most of the B complex, iodine, magnesium, zinc, copper, and sodium. (Duke, Aulik, and Plowman, *Harvard Botanical Museum Leaflets* 24 (6), 1975). These are the elements which must be replaced if you use cocaine.

"Vitamin C, 1,000 mg. A.M. and P.M. (time release), is strongly recommended, along with a stress B complex, 50 mg.," says *Earl Mindell's Vitamin Bible* (Rawson, Wade, N.Y., 1979). "A good multiple-vitamin and mineral tablet as well as a high-potency mineral taken twice daily is also advised." If you have a sudden craving for peanut butter during or after a coke session, it may be a sign that your B vitamins are depleted. The B complex should be taken with food, and metabolizes rapidly, so take more than 50 mg. daily if you're doing a lot of cocaine. The way to gauge this is to keep your piss yellow. Vitamin A should be taken sparingly because it's easy to overdose (nausea, diarrhœa, chills).

Vitamin E, 100 to 400 IU daily, seems to help spruce up your cardiorespiratory system. Acting as a vasodilator and mild diuretic, it lowers blood pressure and helps repair damaged tissues by enriching the blood's oxygen supply. If you smoke anything—tobacco, marijuana, or freebase—take vitamin E to protect your lungs. Also be aware that ferrous sulfate, a form of iron often found in multiple-vitamin formulas, destroys vitamin E. Use a formula that contains iron as ferrous fumarate or gluconate. Learning to use vitamins is almost as tricky as learning to use drugs.

A program of daily exercise, good diet, and vitamins will help flush toxic chemicals from your system and, as a bonus, will make cocaine more effective the next time it is consumed. But if you neglect this healthy regime, coke simply adds to the poisons that accumulate in your system, and makes you feel lower, not higher.

Thirdly, clean your nose without fail after every coke session (not after every toot). The nose is the respiratory system's natural air conditioner. As air flows up through the nostrils and down through the pharynx, larynx, and trachea, it passes over mucous membranes which warm it, and catch foreign particles to purify it, on its way to the lungs. Cocaine when snorted tries to follow the same route but gets dissolved almost instantly on the membranes, entering the blood stream through the many tiny vessels of the membranes. At the same time, cocaine restricts these blood vessels and anesthetizes the cilia which keep the mucous blanket moving back over the membranes. Thus the membranes dry out and stop functioning, leading very quickly to dryness, crusting, and ulceration in your nose. Every time you take a toot you are turning your air conditioner off. Unless you help restore this necessary function, you render yourself susceptible to nagging colds, bacterial infections, and a host of respiratory diseases.

There are two steps to cleaning your nose and reviving your air conditioner. First, make a weak saline solution in a glass with 1/4 teaspoon salt in a cup of warm water. Pinch your thumb and forefinger together and pour a little of this solution over them. Raise this to your nostrils and sniff gently so a tepid salt spray is spread over the membranes inside. Alternatively, pour some into your cupped palm. Close one nostril and inhale through the other until water washes back into your throat. Change nostrils and repeat. You don't need much, and you don't have to go through any contortions like bending your head way back. Commercial nose sprays are pretty rough on nasal passages already irritated by cocaine, and should not be used frequently.

Once your nasal cavity is irrigated, the second step is to lubricate it with vitamin E oil. A natural vitamin E "beauty oil" sold at cosmetics counters is okay for this if it contains only alpha-tocopherol in an organic medium like safflower oil. Or you can open up a capsule of vitamin E with a razor blade. Some people prefer a lanolin-petrolatum ointment of the kind used for diaper rash, but this is too heavy for more than occasional use in the nose.

If your fingers are large, use a cotton swab for the application: most people will find this preferable. You can use the tip of your little finger if it's small, clean, and not jagged. Dab some E oil on the swab or fingertip and *very carefully and slowly* stick it up your nose. *Gently* wiggle it so the oil coats the membranes on all sides. Repeat the procedure in the same nostril, making sure that you lubricate the entire inner rim of the nostril and the little pocket near the tip of your nose. Do the same for the other side, glance in the mirror, smile smugly, say "next time," and go to bed. Don't worry if your nose starts feeling stuffy again: it's your mucous membranes beginning to revive. The tingling in your nose should vanish by the time you fall asleep.

A perforated septum is more often caused by clumsy attempts to clean the nose than by cocaine. The nose needs time to recover from the irritation of any foreign substance put in it. As with cocaine itself, douching and oiling more than every few days may harm your nose—and worse, your sinuses.

If crusting in your nose continues or if you start getting nosebleeds, lay off the cocaine and see your doctor without delay. If you notice any malfunction in your system whatsoever, it could be a warning signal of an oncoming illness and should be checked out by a trusted physician. By having a checkup at the first sign of anything wrong you may avert a real tragedy. Paying attention is the definition of a connoisseur.

Michael R. Aldrich

(Continued from page 52)

to prevent recrystallization of the base in the bowl. Where freebasing is done there is also usually some very flammable solvent; an open flame near such solvents is a potential disaster.

Smoking freebase cocaine in this way is strictly an American phenomenon. Although both pasta and base have been smoked in South America for years, they are much less pure forms of cocaine and are almost always combined with tobacco when smoked. Base is made from pasta (cocaine sulfate) to make crystal (cocaine hydrochloride). Freebase is made from crystal in order to be smoked.

(Continued on page 58)

COKE AND SEX

Since cocaine is widely used as a sex aid, a few words should be said about applying cocaine to the genital organs. A sprinkle of coke on the clitoris or just below the head of the penis will anesthetize the tissues and retard sexual climax. If this is done sparingly and only occasionally it can promote explosive orgasms. However, when cocaine was widely used as a surgical anesthetic around the turn of the century, doctors discovered that the urethra (the tube inside the penis or vulva through which urine is eliminated from the bladder) is very sensitive to cocaine: several patients died from an overdose of cocaine in this area. Don't apply cocaine directly to the hole in the tip of the penis or to the urethral opening between the clitoris and the vaginal orifice in the vulva. And because coke severely dries delicate membranes that must be moist in order to function, don't cover the penis with coke and don't put coke inside the vagina.

Michael R. Aldrich

TREATMENT OF COCAINE OVERDOSE

A cocaine overdose usually happens so fast that nothing can be done about it at home. The symptoms are: giddiness, wooziness, delirium, respiratory depression, Cheyne-Stokes breathing (a pattern whereby breathing builds deeper and deeper to a point, then becomes progressively shallower, with a period of no breathing between cycles), convulsions, and unconsciousness followed by death from respiratory failure. The heart may also stop. Quick action is necessary to save the victim's life. Stay calm, and don't let your fear of arrest prevent you from acting decisively.

Have the victim lie down on his or her back with head lower than body, try to maintain breathing by artificial respiration, and get the victim to a hospital as quickly as possible no matter how embarrassed you are. Call an ambulance if you don't have a car. Be honest with the emergency room people about what drugs the victim has taken, and *bring a small sample* they can analyze if complications set in. Cocaine is so often adulterated that the sample may be necessary to determine what chemicals the victim has ingested.

Do not give the victim more drugs of any kind. There are no real antidotes to cocaine, though the hospital staff may administer intravenous Valium or a short-acting barbiturate to control seizures. The danger here is that downers may cause death by further depressing the cardiorespiratory system. The best "cure" for an overdose is to make sure that it doesn't happen in the first place.

Michael R. Aldrich

There is no such thing as a "bad" drug. People can abuse almost any chemical substance ever invented. Some substances are, however, more subject to abuse than others. For example, although the phenothiazine drugs are central nervous system depressants, they are rarely, if ever, abused; they do not cause a euphoria. On the other hand, central nervous system stimulants such as caffeine, cocaine and amphetamine, and depressants such as barbiturates and alcohol, are frequently abused; they cause euphoria. Our society has chosen alcohol, caffeine and nicotine as euphoriants—though the alcoholic psychoses are certainly not innocuous. We choose our poisons on the basis of tradition, not pharmacology. Societal attitudes determine which drugs are accepted and the extent to which moral qualities are ascribed to chemicals.

Dr. Robert Byck,
Cocaine Papers, 1974.

DOONESBURY April 10, 1980 **by Garry Trudeau**

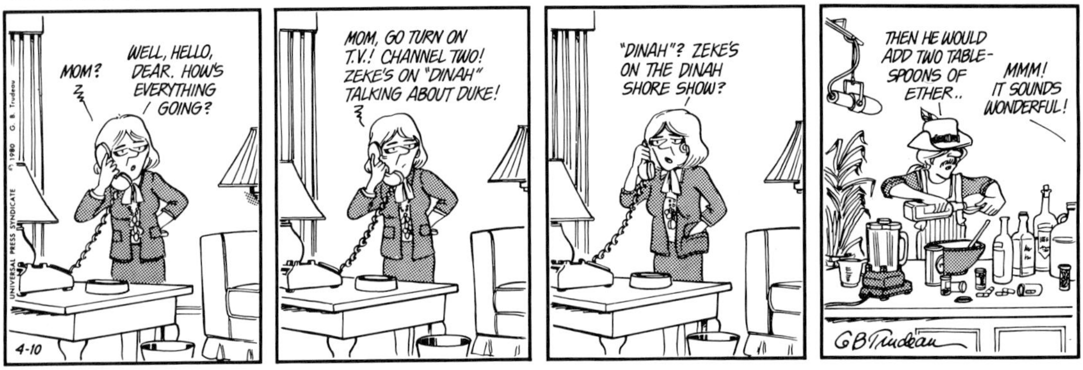
MOM?
WELL, HELLO, DEAR. HOW'S EVERYTHING GOING?
MOM, GO TURN ON T.V.! CHANNEL TWO! ZEKE'S ON "DINAH" TALKING ABOUT DUKE!
"DINAH"? ZEKE'S ON THE DINAH SHORE SHOW?
THEN HE WOULD ADD TWO TABLE-SPOONS OF ETHER..
MMM! IT SOUNDS WONDERFUL!

The first hit is wonderful! It's a feeling of warmth and excitement that starts in your chest, works up through your spine, clear up out the top of your head and while you're holding your breath, it feels as if the cosmos is spinning. It only happens once or twice and you never forget. Every time you do free base you are trying to recapture the unique grace of that first hit and it is just impossible to do so. You're wasting time and energy trying to recapture something you can only remember.

Michael Aldrich (from an interview with Suzanne Knittel for Video West, 1981).

(Continued from page 56)

The smoke which is drawn into the mouth is absorbed into the bloodstream through the lung tissue. This is not only the most direct route to the brain, it is also the most effective means of absorption. For this reason, individual doses of freebase tend to be smaller than with snorting. The effects are more quickly and strongly felt, but are experienced for a shorter period of time.

The attraction of the freebase high is the initial rush, which subsequent tokes rarely recapture. This hardly keeps anyone from trying, and with the comedown in such strong contrast to the rush, an attempt is usually made to maintain the short-lived high by consuming repeated doses of increasing amounts. This often results in binges lasting from several hours to several days. It is very common among freebase users to attempt to balance the extreme high with some type of depressant. Once relaxed, it is even easier to consume freebase in mass quantities.

There is a common misconception among freebasers that the process used to free the base will remove all adulterants leaving only cocaine. Nothing could be further from the truth. There are literally thousands of drugs, both synthetic and naturally occurring, which will convert to freebases along with cocaine. Few if any of these will produce the euphoria which is unique to cocaine, and a few tokes are likely to produce a reaction that the user is not likely to forget.

(Continued on page 60)

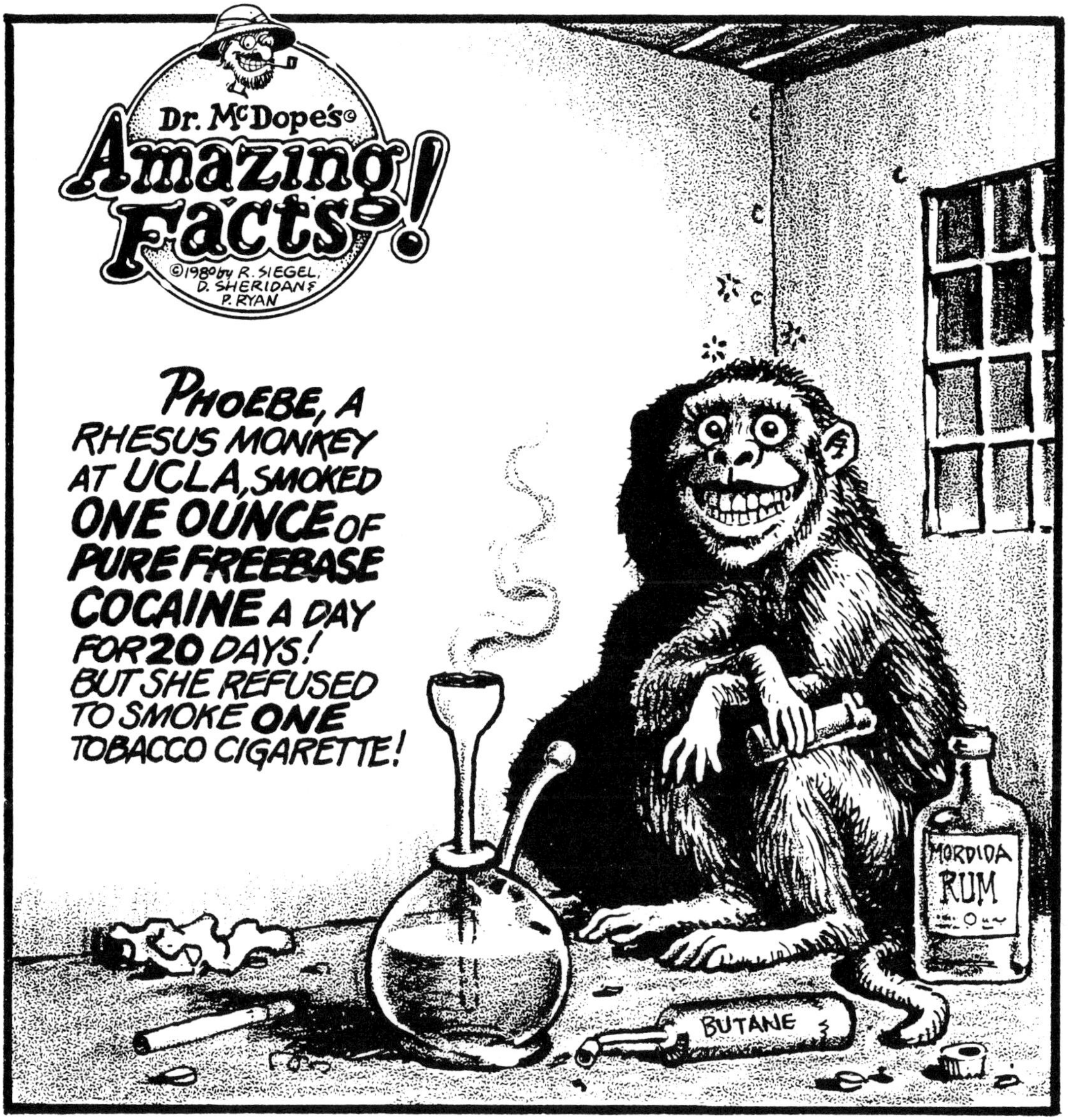
Dr. McDope's©
Amazing Facts!
©1980 by R. SIEGEL, D. SHERIDAN & P. RYAN
PHOEBE, A RHESUS MONKEY AT UCLA, SMOKED ONE OUNCE OF PURE FREEBASE COCAINE A DAY FOR 20 DAYS! BUT SHE REFUSED TO SMOKE ONE TOBACCO CIGARETTE!
MORDIDA RUM
BUTANE

Freebase can induce a very intense compulsive behavioral pattern of compulsive use. You get to the point where freebase is the only thing in your life. You live, die, everything for freebase and in that comes chronic use, lack of sleep, hallucinations, paranoia. If you have any kind of heart problem or are prone to any kind of heart problem, it certainly can freeze your heart. The freebase subculture has permeated every level of society. Freebase has a very debilitating effect on your lungs (and the passage of oxygen in your lungs). People have been known to spit up black phlegm.

Darryl Inaba, M.D. (from an interview with Suzanne Knittel for Video West, 1981).

While there is an abundance of information regarding the effects of cocaine snorting on the nasal membranes, very little is known about the effects of freebase smoke on the lungs. Anyone who has used freebase has no doubt noticed its tendency to recrystallize in the bowl and stem of the pipe which is used. The question must be raised as to whether this recrystallization also occurs in the lungs. It is a common practice to clean the freebase pipe with solvent; the nose is cleaned with salt water. Unfortunately, one cannot apply a similar procedure on the lungs.

The freebase smoker is likely to be confronted with the same psychological problems which face most cocaine users. However, as with the freebase high, they will be more quickly and strongly felt. This is in part due to the vast difference in purity which usually exists between freebase and the street coke from which it came. Pure substances like cocaine are generally more dangerous to consume than a less concentrated form. An obvious analogy is caffeine which exists as a small percentage of the coffee most people drink. The morning cup of coffee is a socially acceptable way to increase alertness, and for most people the side effects are minimal. On the other hand, if we were to consume pure caffeine by snorting or smoking it, overdosage would be much more likely and any side effects would be much more apparent.

The most prevalent danger of freebase consumption is its tendency to totally captivate its user. Chronic users of freebase tend to do little else. To say that freebase is a drug which does not encourage outward communication would be a gross understatement. Freebasers generally use larger quantities of purer cocaine than with any other route of administration. One quarter-ounce, 7 grams, of cocaine hydrochloride converted to freebase is not an uncommon amount to be consumed daily and much larger amounts have been documented.

The author feels a moral responsibility to especially discourage the use of freebase cocaine. While the old saying, "anything in moderation," still holds true, the use of freebase tends to encourage anything *but* moderation.

TWO OPINIONS

The psychic effect of *cocaïnum muriaticum* in doses of 0.05–0.10g consists of exhilaration and lasting euphoria, which does not differ in any way from the normal euphoria of a healthy person. . . . One senses an increase of self-control and feels more vigorous and more capable of work. . . . One is simply normal, and soon finds it difficult to believe that one is under the influence of any drug at all.

Dr. Sigmund Freud, describing a 50 mg. oral dose. *Cocaine Papers,* 1884.

During recent years I have seen among men of science frightful symptoms due to the craving for cocaine. Those who believe they can enter the temple of happiness through this gate of pleasure purchase their momentary delights at the cost of body and soul. They speedily pass through the gate of unhappiness into the night of the abyss.

Dr. Louis Lewin, 1924 quoted in R. Byck, *Cocaine Papers,* 1974.

People who have never shown any prior tendency towards addiction may join hands with chronic users, passing the pipe until the last of it goes up in smoke. Experienced cocaine consumers often stop smoking freebase entirely because of its disastrous effects on the mind, the body, and the pocketbook.

Cocaine is sometimes consumed by injection, which by its very nature is extremely hard on the circulatory system and is possibly a form of suicide. As with freebase,

Heavy cocaine users report a sense that things are crawling on or under their skin—the so-called "cocaine bugs" phenomenon. "But these are pseudohallucinations," says Siegel. "The patients always say it's *as if* there were bugs under their skin. They don't act on a belief that there actually are."

Freebase, on the other hand, *can* stimulate frighteningly real hallucinations. One man in a group of cocaine users Siegel has studied for five years went through four and a quarter ounces of freebase in three days. He became convinced he could see "black antibodies" in his muscle tissue forcing dangerous white worms out of his skin. He examined the antibodies and worms with a thirty-power microscope and, with a needle and tweezers, began removing the "worms" from his flesh and put them in vials for documentation. He brought Siegel ten vials of "worms." There was nothing in the vials but dried human tissue. This was a genuine paranoid hallucination, and the man's girlfriend, who had only smoked three-quarters of an ounce of freebase over the same period, was seeing the worms, too.

Charles Perry, *Rolling Stone,* 1980.

the effects are strongly felt and extremely short lived. As with freebase, this usually leads to stronger and more frequent doses. The result can be damaged veins, skin abscesses, and hepatitis, in addition to the constant risk of overdose. The problem may be further compounded by the presence of impurities and/or adulterants which are usually present in street cocaine. Where non-water soluble substances are involved, the results can be fatal.

A less common method of consuming cocaine consists of dissolving the hydrochloride in water or other suitable liquid and drinking it. This is the method Sigmund Freud himself used for consuming cocaine, but when taken this way most of the cocaine must pass through the stomach before getting into the bloodstream. Some authors think most of the cocaine is broken down in the stomach, while others disagree; it might depend on how acid the stomach is and how long it takes the cocaine to get through the stomach.

How do people like this producer afford the thousands of dollars necessary to keep performers supplied with coke? The simplest way is to add the expense to the cost of the production. "Money for drugs is always there. You hide it in the budget under 'miscellaneous' or 'food' or 'entertainment'." Another producer disclosed his technique: "I hide it under 'props' in the budget. Who checks?" One studio head joked about his creative bookkeeping. "There are three kinds of costs: above-the-line, below-the-line and cocaine-line," he said.

Frank Swertlow, in *T.V. Guide*, Feb. 28, 1981.

Cocaine and Economics

A consumer might think about this: coke goes for \$75–150 per gram, and \$1800–3000 an ounce (28 grams). Instead of buying one gram of cocaine he could:

See 30 movies
Buy 15 record albums
Play 1000 games of pinball, or
Buy one ounce of sinsemilla.

The cost of two grams of coke could get him:

15 cases of Heinekens
4 good pairs of shoes, or
5 shares of A.T.&T.

If the consumer does 2 grams a month he could be living in a much nicer apartment. Three could be a color television. Four grams could be a weekend in Hawaii. Seven could be a Sony Betamax. Looking at it from a less selfish angle, the money spent on cocaine could provide a foster child with milk, food, toys, medical, and dental care for an entire year. The consumer can have any of these things or get high for twenty minutes. (Adapted and updated from Paul Slansky, *New Times Magazine*, July 22, 1977.)

Cocaine and the Law

The fact that cocaine possession and sale is illegal has not deterred thousands of regular users. Very few people have had to deal with the legal implications of cocaine use, and most users remain unaware of the legal penalties which exist. Nowhere is this more true than in foreign countries which are visited by thousands of American tourists each year. While the leniency of the law may vary with circumstances and connections, a basic understanding and familiarity with the law should be clear in the minds of all cocaine users.

The statutes listed on the following pages are subject to change; they are correct as of January 1, 1981.

There is considerable variation in the form of statutes from state to state so for details the particular state statute should be consulted. This table illustrates the great difference in penalties; terms range from 90 days to 20 years for first conviction for possession and longer terms for sale.

In general the class of crime can be related to the length of term. A felony is a crime for which the punishment can be imprisonment for more than one year and a misdemeanor ranges from one day to one year. Felony terms are usually served in prison or penitentiary (state institution) and misdemeanor terms are served in city or county jails.

Although the cocaine laws were written as if they were a tax measure they, like the marijuana laws, appeared to be written primarily for the purpose of protecting public health and morality. Yet the laws forbidding the use of marijuana and cocaine have been no more successful in that aim than was Prohibition . . . but as long as the laws are in conflict with widely accepted practices, society can expect some of its most productive citizens to be caught in the crossfire.

Editorial,
Oakland Tribune,
Feb. 5, 1981.

OVERVIEW OF COCAINE LAWS AND PENALTIES FOR THE 50 STATES

STATE	VIOLATION	QUANTITY	# of Offenses	TERM (Years)		FINE (Dollars)
ALABAMA	possession or sale	any	1	2-15	and poss.	max. $25,000
	possesion or sale to a minor (under 18)	any	1	4-30	and poss.	max. $50,000
		any	2 or more	twice above		twice above
ALASKA	possession or sale	any	1	2-10	and	max. $5,000
		any	2	10-20	and	$7,500
		any	3	20-40	and	$10,000
	sale to person under 21	any	1	10-30	and	$5,000-$10,000
		any	2	15-30	and	max. $25,000
		any	3	life		
ARIZONA	possession	any	1	2-10		
		any	2	5-20		
		any	3	15-life		
	narcotics for sale	any	1	5-15		
		any	2	min. 10		
		any	3	min. 15		
	import and transport of narcotic drugs; sales and traffic in narcotic drugs	any	1	5-life		
		any	2	10-life		
		any	3	15-life		
	inducing minors tc violate narcotic drug laws	any	1	10-life, parole after 5		
		any	2	10-life, parole after 10		
		any	3	15-life		
ARKANSAS	possession	2 grams	1	2-10		
		2 grams	2	3-15		
		2 grams	4 or more	10-20		
	sale or possession with intent to sell	more than 2 grams	1	5-50 or life		
		more than 2 grams	2	10-50 or life		
	(possession of more than 2 grams is considered presumptive evidence of intent to sell)	more than 2 grams	4 or more	min. 50, max. life		
CALIFORNIA	possession	any	1	2-10		
		any	2	5-20		
		any	3	15-life		
	possession for sale	any	1	5-15		
		any	2	min. 10		
		any	3	min. 15		
	transportation, sale, giving away, etc.	any	1	5-life		
		any	2	10-life		
		any	3	15-life		
COLORADO	possession and sale	any	1	2-15	and	max. $10,000
		any	2	5-20	and	max. $10,000
		any	3	10-30	and	max. $10,000
	possession for sale and sell or induce another person to unlawfully use	any	1	10-20		
		any	2	15-30		
		any	3 or more	20-40		

CONNECTICUT	possession	any any any	1 2 3 or more	max. 7 max. 15 max. 25	and/or and/or and/or	max. $3,000 max. $5,000 max. $10,000
	sale	less than 1 ounce less than 1 ounce more than 1 ounce	1 2 or more	5-20 10-25 min. 5-25, max. life		
DELAWARE	possession	any		max. 5	and	max. $3,000
	sale or possession with intent to sell	any		30, no parole	and	$25,000-$100,000
DISTRICT OF COLUMBIA	possession or sale	any any	1 2 or more	max. 1 max. 10	and/or and/or	$100-$1,000 $500-$5,000
FLORIDA	possession	any any	1 2 or more	max. 5 max. 10	and/or	max. $5,000
	sale or possession with intent to sell	any any	1 2 or more	max. 15 max. 30	and/or	max. $10,000
GEORGIA	possession	any any	1 2 or more	2-15 5-30		
	sale	any any	1 2 or more	5-30 life		
	possession and/or sale (trafficking in cocaine)	28-200 grams 200-400 grams 400 grams or more		min. mandatory 5 min. mandatory 7 min. mandatory 15	and and and	$50,000 $100,000 $250,000
HAWAII	promoting dangerous drug/3rd degree	possesion less than 1/8 ounce	1 or 2 3 or more	max. 5 extended terms		
	promoting dangerous drug/2nd degree	possession 1/8 ounce or more; distirbution of any amount	1 or 2 3 or more	max. 10 extended terms		
	promoting dangerous drug/1st degree	possession over 1 oz.; distribution over 1/8 oz.; distribution of any amount to minor 3 years younger	1 or 2 3 or more	max. 20 extended terms		
IDAHO	possession	any		max. 3	and/or	max. $7,000
	possession with intent to sell or sale	any		max. life	and/or	max. $25,000
ILLINOIS	possession	under 30 grams over 30 grams		1-3 4-15	and and	max. $15,000 max. $100,000
	possession with intent to sell or sale	under 30 grams over 30 grams		3-7 6-30	and and	max. $25,000 max. $200,000
INDIANA	possession	under 10 grams over 10 grams		fixed 2, ±2 for circumstances fixed 5, ±3 for circumstances		
	sale or possession with intent to sell	under 10 grams over 10 grams		fixed 10, +10 or -4 for circumstances fixed 30, +20 or -10 for circumstances		

continued

Overview of Cocaine Laws (continued)

STATE	VIOLATION	QUANTITY	# of Offenses	TERM (Years)		FINE (Dollars)
IOWA	possession	any		max. 1	and/or	max. $1,000
	sale or possession with intent to sell	any		max. 10	and/or	max. $5,000
KANSAS	possession and/or sale	any		indeterminate min. 1-3, max. 10	and/or	max. $5,000
KENTUCKY	possession	any	1	1-5	and/or	$3,000-$5,000
		any	2 or more	5-10	and/or	$5,000-$10,000
	sale	any	1	5-10	and/or	$5,000-$10,000
		any	2 or more	10-20	and/or	$10,000-$20,000
LOUISIANA	possession	under 28 grams		with or without hard labor max. 5	and poss.	max. $5,000
		28-200 grams		hard labor, 5-30	and	min. $50,000
		200-400 grams		hard labor, 10-30	and	min. $100,000
		400 grams or more		hard labor, 15-30	and	min. $250,000
	sale, manufacture or possession with intent to sell	any		hard labor, 5-30	and poss.	max. $15,000
MAINE	possession	any		definite max. 1		
	sale or possession with intent to sell	any		definite max. 10		
MARYLAND	possession, manufacture or sale	any		max. 20	and poss.	max. $25,000
MASSACHU-SETTS	possession or sale	any		max. 10 state prison, max. 2½ jail or house of correction	and/or	max. $20,000
MICHIGAN	possession	less than 50 grams		max. 4	and/or	max. $2,000
		50-225 grams		10-20 or life probation		
		225-650 grams		20-30		
		650 grams or more		life		
	sale, manufacture, possession with intent to sell	less than 50 grams		max. 20	and/or	max. $25,000
		50-225 grams		10-20 or life probation		
		225-650 grams		20-30		
		650 grams or more		life		
MINNESOTA	possession	any		max. 5	and/or	max. $5,000
	sale	any	1	max. 15	and/or	max. $25,000
		any	2 or more	min. 1, max. 30	and/or	max. $50,000
MISSISSIPPI	possession	any	1	max. 3	and/or	max. $3,000
		any	2 or more	may double above	and/or	may double above
	sale	any	1	min. 3, max. 30	and poss.	max. $30,000
			2 or more	may double above	and poss.	may double above

MISSOURI	possession	any any any	1 2 3	max. 20 5-life 10-life		
	sale	any any	1 2	5-life 10-life		
MONTANA	possession	any		max. 5		
	possession with intent to sell	any		max. 20		
	sale	any any any	1 2 3	1-life 5-life 10-life		
NEBRASKA	possession	any		max. 5, min. none	and/or	$10,000
	sale	any		max. 20, min. 1	and/or	$25,000
NEVADA	possession	any any any	1 2 3	1-6 1-10 1-20	and poss. and poss. and poss.	max. $5,000 max. $10,000 max. $20,000
	sale	any any any	1 2 3	life or definite 1-20 life or definite 5-20 life or definite min. 15	and poss. and poss. and poss.	max. $20,000 max. $20,000 max. $20,000
NEW HAMPSHIRE	possession	any any	1 2 or more	max. 7 max. 15		
	sale	any		max. 15, extended terms for certain circumstances		
NEW JERSEY	possession	**A.** less than 1 oz. including adulterants or 1 oz. or more with there being included less than 3.5 grams of the pure free base		max. 5	and poss.	max. $15,000
		B. 1 oz. or more including adulterants or dilutants provided there are included at least 3.5 grams of the pure free base		max. 7	and poss.	max. $15,000
	sale, possession with intent to sell	same as **A** above same as **B** above		max. 12 max. life	and poss. and poss.	max. $25,000 max. $25,000
NEW MEXICO	possession	any		1½	and poss.	max. $5,000
	trafficking (sale, possession with intent to sell)	any any	1 2	9 18	and poss. and poss.	max. $10,000 max. $15,000

continued

Overview of Cocaine Laws (continued)

STATE	VIOLATION	QUANTITY	# of Offenses	TERM (Years)		FINE (Dollars)
NEW YORK	possession	less than 1/8 oz.		max. 1	and/or	max. $1,000
		1/8 oz.-1/2 oz.		indeterminate 1-15		
		½ oz.-2 oz.		indeterminate 1-25		
		2 oz.-4 oz.		indeterminate 3-life		
		4 oz. or more		indeterminate 15-life		
	sale	less than ½ ounce		indeterminate 1-25		
		½ oz.-2 oz.		indeterminate 3-life		
		2 oz. or more		indeterminate 15-life		
NORTH CAROLINA	possession	less than 1 gram		max. 2	and/or	max. $3,000
		1 gram or more		max. 5	and/or	max. $5,000
	sale	any		max. 10	and/or	max. $10,000
NORTH DAKOTA	possession	any		max. 5	and/or	$5,000
	sale, manufacture, possession with intent to sell	any		max. 20	and/or	$10,000
OHIO	possession	any	1	½-5		max. $2,500
		any	2 or more	1-10		max. $5,000
	trafficking	less than 10 grams	1	1-10		max. $5,000
		less than 10 grams	2 or more	2-15		max. $7,500
OKLAHOMA	possession	any	1	2-10		
		any	2 or more	4-20		
	sale, manufacture, possession with intent to sell	any	1	5-20	and	max. $20,000
		any	2 or more	twice the above	and	twice the above
OREGON	possession	any		max. 5		
	sale	any		max. 10	and poss.	max. $2,500 or max. that of gain by the crime
PENNSYLVANIA	possession	any		max. 3	or	max. $5,000
	sale	any	1	max. 15	or	max. $250,000
		any	2 or more	may double above		may double above
RHODE ISLAND	possession	any		max. 3	and/or	max. $1,000
	sale	any		max. life		
SOUTH CAROLINA	possession	up to 10 grains	1	max. 2	and/or	max. $5,000
		up to 10 grains	2	max. 3	and/or	max. $5,000
		up to 10 grains	3 or more	max. 4	and/or	max. $10,000
	sale, manufacture, possession with intent to sell	any	1	max. 15	and/or	max. $25,000
		any	2	5-30	and/or	max. $50,000
		any	3 or more	15-30	and/or	max. $50,000
	(possession of more than 10 grains is presumptive of the intent to sell)					

SOUTH DAKOTA	possession	any		2	and/or	$2,000
	sale, manufacture, possession with intent to sell	any		10	and poss.	$10,000
TENNESSEE	possession	any any any	1 2 3 or more	max. 1 1-2 2-3	and/or	max. $1,000
	sale	less than 30 grams 30 grams or more		4-10 10-life	and poss. and poss.	max. $15,000 max. $200,000
	"habitual drug offender"	multiple violations		10-life	and poss.	max. $200,000
TEXAS	possession	any		2-20	and poss.	max. $10,000
	sale, manufacture, possession with intent to deliver	any		life or 5-99		
UTAH	possession	any any any	1 2 3 or more	max. ½ max. 1 max. 5	and/or and/or	max. $299 max. $1,000
	sale or possession with intent to sell	any		max. 15	and/or	max. $15,000
VERMONT	possession		1 2 or more	max. 1 max. 2 + 1 day	and/or and/or	max. $1,000 max. $3,000
	possession with intent to sell or possession of more than 500 milligrams			max. 3	and/or	max. $3,000
	possession with intent to sell same for a consideration or in an amount of more than 1 gram			max. 5	and/or	max. $5,000
	sale, manufacture and dispersing any quantity			max. 5	and/or	max. $10,000
	sale to person under 18 years old			max. 25	and/or	max. $25,000
VIRGINIA	possession	any		1-10	and/or	max. $1,000
	sale or possession with intent to sell	any		5-40	and	max. $25,000
WASHINGTON	possession	any		max. 5	and/or	max. $10,000
	sale or possession with intent to sell	any		max. 10	and/or	max. $25,000
WEST VIRGINIA	possession	any		¼-½	and/or	max. $1,000
	sale or possession with intent to sell	any		1-15	and/or	max. $15,000
WISCONSIN	possession	any any	1 2 or more	max. 1 max. 2	and/or and/or	max. $5,000 max. $10,000
	sale or possession with intent to sell	any		max. 15	and/or	max. $25,000
WYOMING	possession	any any	1-2 3 or more	max. ½ max. 5	and/or and/or	max. $1,000 max. $5,000
	sale or possession with intent to sell	any		max. 20	and/or	max. $25,000

Chapter Five

Adulterants

Some people argue that cocaine cut with relatively harmless materials is safer to use than pure cocaine. This is a myth based on either (a) the belief that cocaine is a highly toxic, physiologically addictive drug, or (b) the notion that the effects of pure cocaine are too powerful for most people to handle. Neither claim has any basis in fact. Except in very large doses, cocaine is rapidly detoxified by the liver and it is a mild euphoric stimulant, not a powerful one.

Richard Ashley,
High Times, 1979.

As the price of illicit cocaine continues to rise, it becomes increasingly likely that one or more persons in the trade hierarchy will attempt to increase his profits by cutting the cocaine with a substance of lesser value. Although it is the consumer who will ultimately be cheated, he may often encourage adulteration by failing to set and maintain a qualitative standard by which to judge each purchase. In fact, cocaine is often adulterated in order to lower the selling price in accordance with buyer criteria. Many unaware consumers stubbornly cling to the belief that a $100 gram which is 50% adulterant is a better value than a $150 gram which is untouched.

These days it is extremely rare for illicit cocaine to reach the United States in pure, unadulterated form. This is often due to intentional deletion of steps in the refining process, steps which could decrease the yield by eliminating organic impurities. The result is a higher yield of cruder cocaine base which rarely exceeds 50% in purity. While it is unadulterated, it is still very far from pure.

When this crude cocaine is converted to the hydrochloride form, the processor will often add an extreme excess of hydrochloric acid in order to speed up the reaction and maintain a high yield. The extra acid often results in some decomposition of the cocaine molecule into benzoylecgonine and ecgonine. This may be easily detected by the odor of wintergreen caused by the formation of methyl benzoate from the decomposition products.

Adulteration at the source is accomplished by several means in addition to forcing a maximum yield from the leaves. There do exist fields of coca which were formerly considered worthless for cocaine production due to the virtual nonexistence of cocaine in the leaves. However, base made from these leaves may be combined with "good base" in order to increase the weight.

Synthetic local anesthetics, especially lidocaine, may be obtained over the counter in Venezuela and Colombia. When lidocaine is added during crystallization, and its amount limited to 25% or less, it is very difficult to detect. Of course, once a 25% cut is successful, the amount is likely to increase in proportion to the greed which motivates it. While other synthetic local anesthetics are often found in illicit cocaine, only lidocaine is readily available in South America. It is therefore logical to assume that a lidocaine cut was added close to the source whereas other synthetics may have been added a little closer to home.

Once the cocaine has reached the United States, it becomes impossible to increase the weight by forcing a higher yield from the leaves. The cocaine is now in the hands of salesmen to whom adulteration may be the only means of increasing the profits. In order to accomplish this, the cocaine and an appropriate adulterant may be reduced to liquids, combined, and reconstituted together in solid form. Often, this is done with some form of **mannitol**, a mild baby laxative which is probably the most common cut used in the United States. Mannitol ("Mannite") is a white crystalline powder which is cheap and easy to get. As "the accepted cocaine cut," it has been advertised in several paraphernalia trade magazines and sold in "head shops." It is by far the least harmful of the more

Most people don't know what they're blowing anyway—they know what they've been buying. You offer them pure and they won't meet your price—they say it's shit because it doesn't look like what they're used to. So you hit it with some borax and they pay your price. But that takes time. After you unload most of it at an honest price, then you can fuck around with what's left for the sucker trade.

Moses Wellfleet, coke dealer, in R. Sabbag, *Snow Blind,* 1976.

common adulterants in terms of its toxicity and its effect on the cocaine. Regardless of its benign qualities, to be sold mannitol as cocaine is to be cheated.

Lactose and **sucrose** are two sugars which are found in adulterated cocaine almost as often as mannitol. They are quite easily obtained, very inexpensive, and relatively harmless. They will, however, dull the appearance of the cocaine, cause post-nasal drip, and crust up the nose.

Inositol is a B vitamin which is sold in health food stores. It is a relatively harmless substance when consumed knowingly, but as a cocaine cut it may be extremely irritating to the nasal passages. It is also very easy to detect in most of the tests outlined in the testing section. Inositol is sold as a white crystalline powder or as needle-shaped crystals.

Caffeine is becoming the most widely used stimulant to adulterate cocaine. It is sold over the counter at chemical supply stores and comes as a small percentage of the ingredients in stimulants like "No Doz." Caffeine, like cocaine, is an alkaloid. It is to coffee what cocaine is to coca. Unlike cocaine, however, caffeine clogs up the nose and irritates the nasal membranes.

Amphetamine or "speed" is a stimulant less commonly used to adulterate cocaine. It is much stronger than caffeine and is usually used to restore the buzz to overly adulterated cocaine. Speed is actually quite popular in its own right, but it is not cocaine, and can be purchased as speed for half the price.

Quinine, though one of the most detrimental of all cocaine cuts, is still widely used. Quinine can produce a reaction in the body quite separate from cocaine. The mood may become somewhat depressed. It can cause ringing in the ears, impaired vision, and can lead to nausea and headache. Its effect on the nasal membranes can be severe irritation from frequent use. Quinine is often used to adulterate heroin, and can be fatal when injected or even snorted.

(Continued on page 74)

FREQUENCY OF APPEARANCE OF ADULTERANTS IN COCAINE

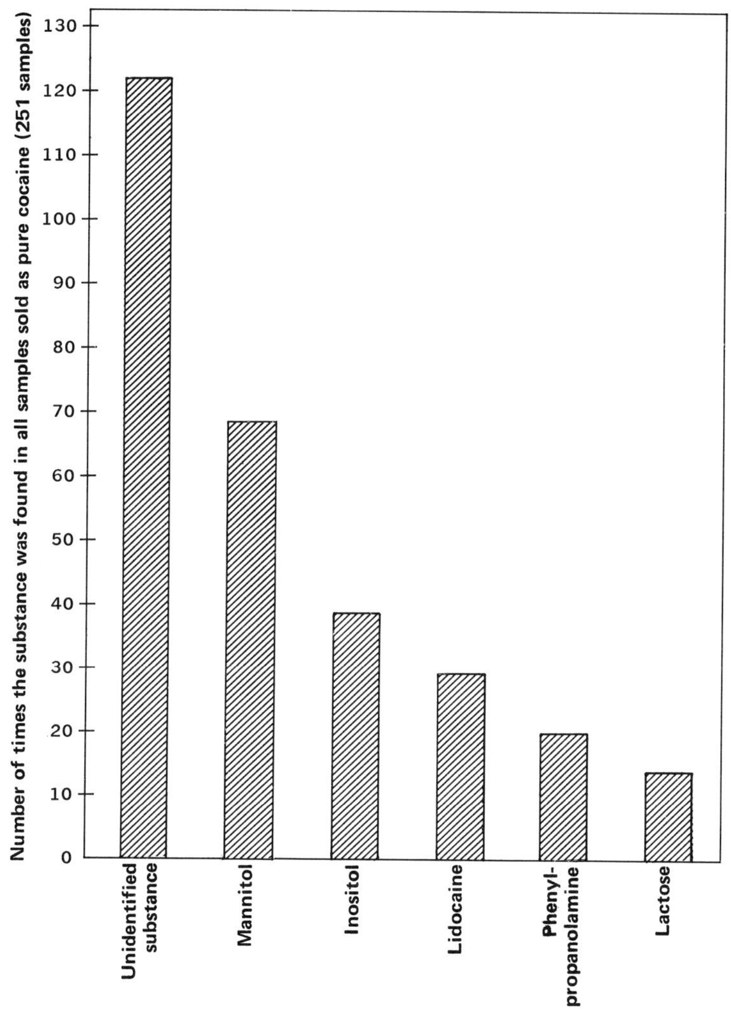

Of 251 samples, 81 were not adulterated (approx. 68% were adulterated).

(Data from PharmChem Laboratories. Samples sold in the U.S. as pure cocaine during January and February in 1981.)

The most common of the active adulterants are the synthetic local anesthetics. These include but are not limited to **lidocaine, procaine, tetracaine, benzocaine,** and **butacaine.** Since cocaine is also a local anesthetic, these synthetics will simulate some of the effects of cocaine and are available at a much lower price. When properly combined, cocaine cut with a synthetic can be very difficult to detect by any street test, and just as difficult to remove using simple purification techniques. One of the most discernable differences between cocaine and lidocaine, for example, is that lidocaine does not produce euphoria. Cocaine alone possesses this quality. Lidocaine has a more pronounced bitter taste, producing almost immediate numbing and lasting longer than cocaine anesthesia. While only tetracaine is of higher toxicity than cocaine, all of the synthetics will produce a state of mind which is somewhat hazy as compared to the clarity of cocaine.

The adulterants listed above are by far the most common.* However, there are very few substances which have not been used to adulterate cocaine at one time or another. The consumer can best protect himself by having a sound knowledge of cocaine, applying varied testing procedures, and above all, using common sense. If the consumer is aware of the reaction of cocaine to tests and upon ingestion, it will be logical to assume that an unknown reaction is caused by an adulterant.

---

* Phenylpropanolamine is a compound which is increasing in popularity as an adulterant for cocaine. In early 1981 it was the fourth most frequently identified adulterant, according to Pharm Chem Laboratories. It is the main ingredient in many non-prescription diet pills and overdoses can produce nervousness, sleeplessness, and dizziness. The melting point of the hydrochloride is 190–194°C., the base 101–101.5°C., for cocaine these values are 195° and 98°C., so if only the melting point above were considered, it could pass for cocaine. This is another example of the value of using a number of tests on a sample.

Chapter Six

Testing

Cocaine testing involves somewhat more than a knowledge of procedures. The tester must develop a feel for analyzing results and applying common sense. While the mechanics of most tests are actually quite simple, the interpretation of the results is much more complex.

A practical approach to testing takes into consideration the location and circumstances surrounding each testing situation.* Very few buyers of illicit cocaine will be testing at the request of the seller, and seldom if ever will this be under laboratory conditions.

Many cocaine dealers, especially those who claim to have knowledge of the origin or purity of the merchandise, will interpret testing as a lack of faith in their integrity.

* A number of chemical tests which give a color reaction with cocaine are available but are not included in this book. The experience of regular consumers is that samples usually do contain cocaine so other concerns become primary. Is it cut with something unpleasant (like quinine), and what is the percent purity? Converting a bit of the sample to cocaine base and weighing it gives an estimate of the percent purity and other tests can detect quinine (the solubility tests). The CRC publication edited by Mulé has excellent detailed discussions of color reaction tests; the book is currently hard to find in bookstores but available in many libraries.

While this may in fact be the case, this interpretation does not make it any easier to accomplish the original intention, that of testing the cocaine. Besides, a negative attitude towards testing does not necessarily indicate dishonesty. Many sellers do not have the time to let each gram buyer run a series of tests, *especially* if it requires an effort on their part to comply.

Know what you intend to do and how you intend to do it, and be confident in your right to examine the merchandise before buying.

—David Lee

The seasoned consumer takes these factors into consideration and has with him the necessary materials to perform the tests in order to lessen the inconvenience to the seller. A small portable testing kit with which the consumer is familiar is used for this purpose.

A common seller's response to a desire to test the cocaine is to offer a small taste as proof of its quality. A polite refusal to use the cocaine prior to testing should only strengthen the consumer's position and may well be interpreted by the seller as proof of the buyer's sincerity. It should be noted that consumption of cocaine prior to testing often effects the interpretation of the results. A cocaine dealer always seems more trustworthy after turning a prospective buyer on to a free snort, and the desire for another often hastens testing procedures or even eliminates them. Consumer willpower to abstain is important here, at least until the tests have been completed.

On Location

Let's assume that the buyer has arrived at the seller's house to purchase a gram of cocaine which is of unknown quality. Since the seller is likely to be using the same coke he is selling, the atmosphere surrounding him (the vibes) may provide the first indication of its quality. His state of mind may well tell how the same cocaine will affect the buyer. If, by chance, the seller is not using the same cocaine he is selling, this should also say something about the quality.

It would be unusual for the buyer to be shown more than the gram he is buying or to see the gram weighed, but should the opportunity arise, there are two good reasons to take advantage of it. The first thing looked for will be the proportion of pieces to duff (powder). How does this compare to that in the gram being purchased? If the seller shows a preference for either, it is likely that they are not the same. (Most adulterants which are mixed in without reconstitution will be found in the duff.) If the seller is indiscriminate, showing no preference for either, it may mean that there is no difference.

The second reason has to do with odor. A large amount of illicit cocaine which has not changed containers recently will give off a more distinguishable odor than a newly weighed gram in a paper bindle. High quality illicit cocaine has little odor, and a recent change of containers may make it falsely seem odorless.

There are two distinguishable scents which are found in illicit cocaine. A sweet smell reminiscent of wintergreen is very common. Its presence usually indicates that some of the cocaine has decomposed. This odor is usually accompanied by an excess of hydrochloric acid and an extreme oiliness in the cocaine. A dusty or musty smell may indicate the presence of an abnormal amount of cocamine. This type of cocaine is usually more opaque in appearance with less of a tendency to form flakelike crystals.

More often than not, the gram being purchased will have been prepackaged and preweighed. Proper etiquette calls for the consumer to make known his intention to test the merchandise and offer to pay for any cocaine used in the process. The bindle is not even opened until this has been made clear. If for some reason this is unacceptable to the seller, the buyer may suggest that the product be tested at the buyer's home and returned should the quality or weight be unsatisfactory.

Sensory Examination

A close sensory examination is not only free but often proves to be quite revealing and informative. The idea is to take a good look at the gram, paying attention to the volume, density, color, and crystallinity. Pure cocaine is very light and fluffy: a gram will more than fill a standard size bindle; screened it will fill a 2-milliliter bottle. Denser substances, whether natural or added adulterants, will greatly decrease the volume. Pure cocaine hydrochloride is a very white crystalline substance. Its sparkle is reminiscent of diamonds. Does the propective gram fit this description? If not, the cause is most often poor refining or adulteration. Is the cocaine appealing? There can be no demeaning the importance of aesthetics to most connoisseurs of cocaine. Aesthetics (whether in cocaine, music, art, or other endeavors) often play an important part in the lives of discerning cocaine users.

A clean, dry razor blade or knife is used to pick through the gram. If any sticks to the blade, the cocaine is not dry. While this does not necessarily indicate adulteration, moisture adds weight which is not cocaine. It can also make it difficult to consume.

A small amount of powdered cocaine is placed on the index finger and rubbed into the skin with the thumb in a circular motion. Pure cocaine disappears into the skin quickly and cleanly, leaving just a trace of oiliness on the skin. It does not feel gritty or greasy.

A small amount of cocaine is placed on the tip of the tongue. High quality cocaine has a slightly bitter, almost medicinal, taste. Numbing is not immediate as with synthetics and will take a few minutes to be felt. There is no sweetness to the taste, nor is it extremely bitter. The sweet taste is usually attributable to some kind of sugar cut, while an extremely bitter taste is usually caused by one of the less active alkaloids like cocamine or hygrine or one of several adulterants. Whatever the variation, the important thing to be remembered is that cocaine has almost no taste at all.

As with all tests, the sensory examination is dependent on previous experience with the real thing. An estimation of quality is difficult without a reference point, and many consumers have never had the opportunity to examine high quality illicit cocaine. This chapter will therefore focus on the reaction of this type of cocaine to various tests. These results will then be compared to results of tests done on the same cocaine to which some common adulterants have been added.

The Methyl Benzoate Test

It seems logical to begin the more objective testing by confirming or denying the presence of cocaine. This may seem rather basic, but it has become more and more common to encounter supposed cocaine which actually has no cocaine in it whatsoever. Cocaine gives a positive test but is not the only chemical that does; however, a negative test means that no cocaine is present.

The test is based on the principle that in the presence of a strong alkali and absolute methanol, cocaine will decompose and a reaction forming methyl benzoate will take place. A positive reaction may be easily recognized by the smell of wintergreen.

To perform the test, a small amount of the cocaine is placed in a dry teaspoon. One drop of a mixture of absolute methanol and sodium hydroxide* is added to the teaspoon and allowed to cover the cocaine. After the methanol has evaporated and the spoon is dry, the sweet smell of wintergreen will be present. This test works well with even a minute quantity of cocaine. If the results are negative (and the test was done correctly) there is no point in further testing. If positive, the next test is done.

Pieces and Duff

It is quite common for cocaine to be adulterated by mixing it with a cheap cut and putting both substances through a coarse screen. Some pieces of cocaine are usually left intact to make it appear as though it has never been touched. To check out this possibility, a sample from the

(Continued on page 87)

---

* Methanol/Sodium hydroxide solution. One gram of NaOH is dissolved in 20 milliliters absolute methanol. Kept tightly stoppered it will keep for months. (Sodium hydroxide is a dangerous caustic.)

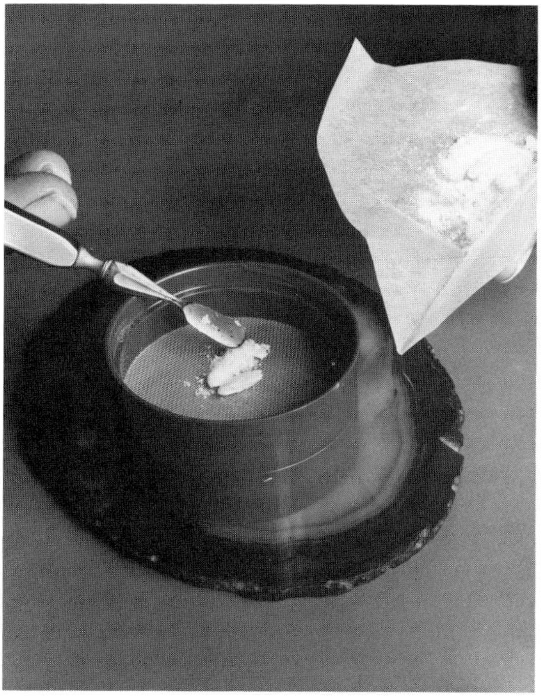

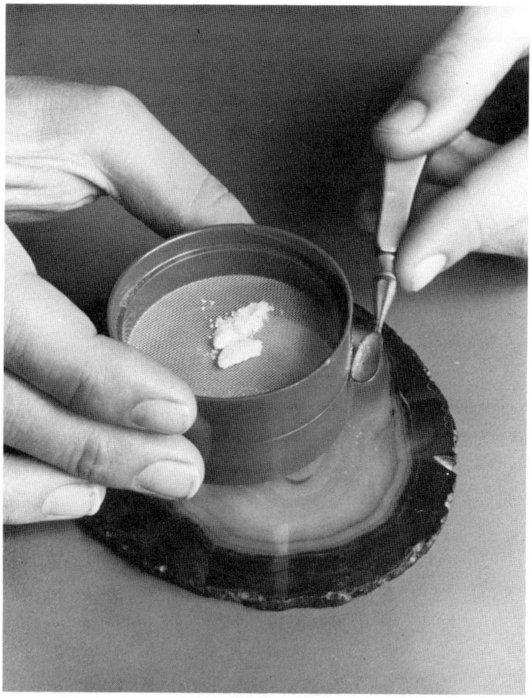

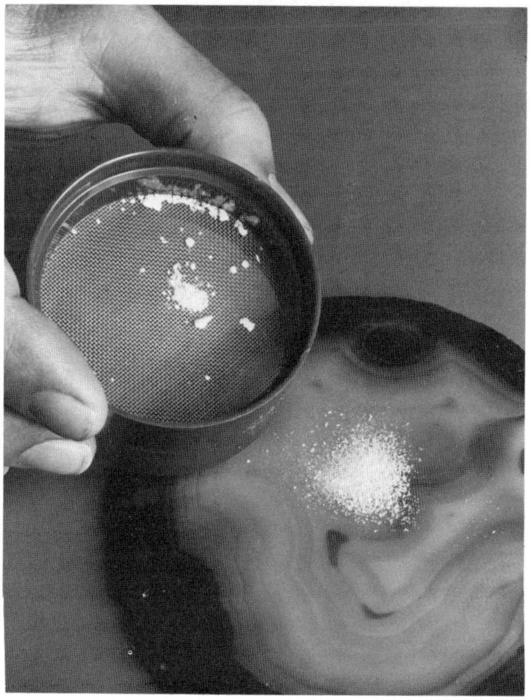

clockwise from top left:

1. The sample is placed on a coarse screen.

2. The screen is lightly tapped.

3. The pieces remain on the screen, while the duff passes through.

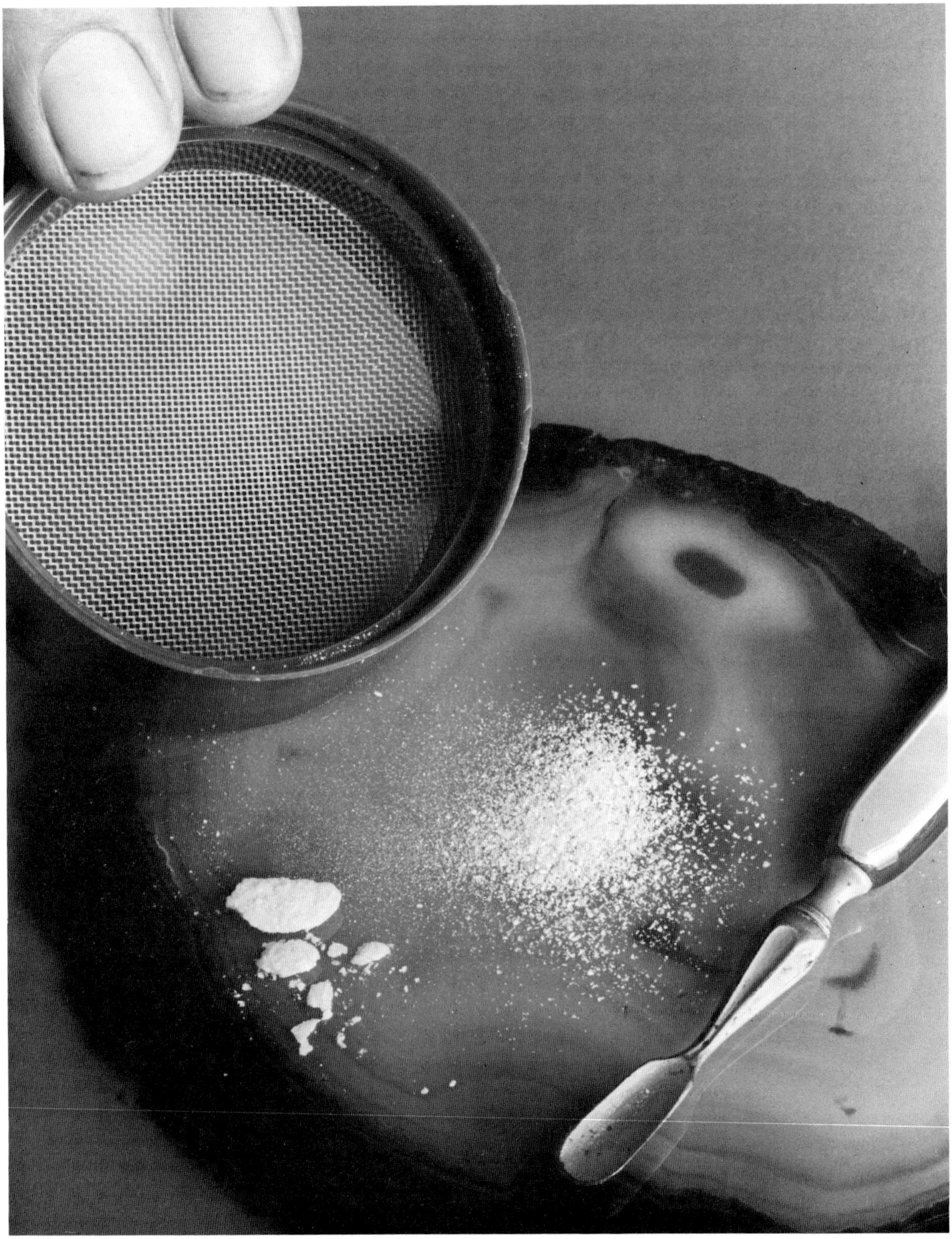

4. The result: duff and pieces separated for comparison.

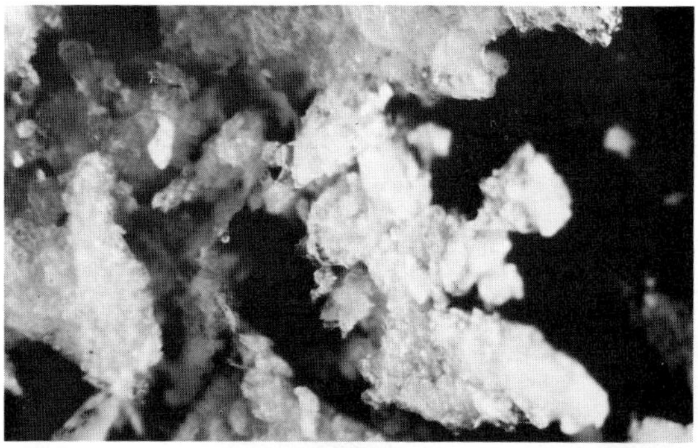

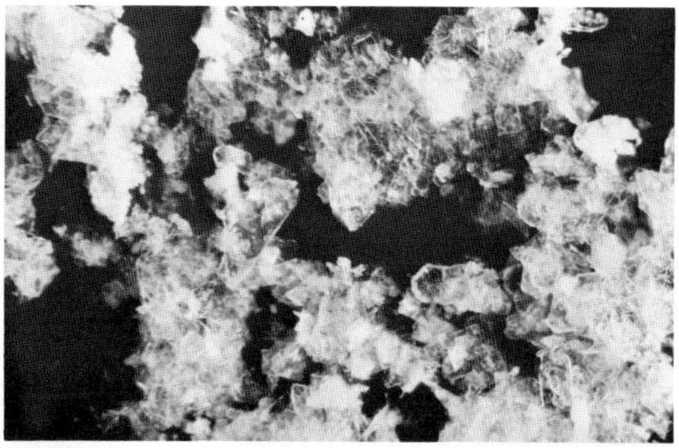

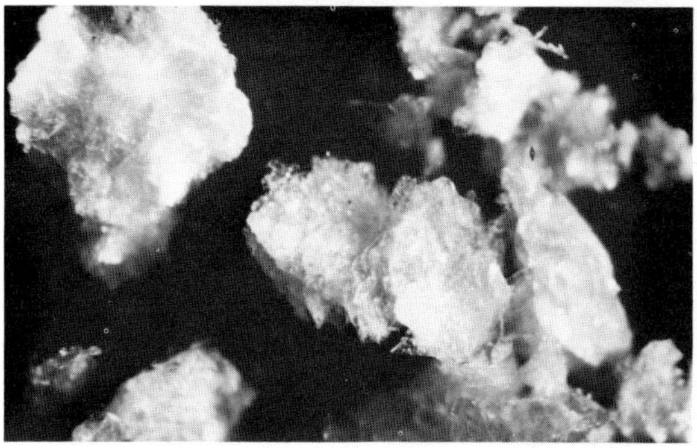

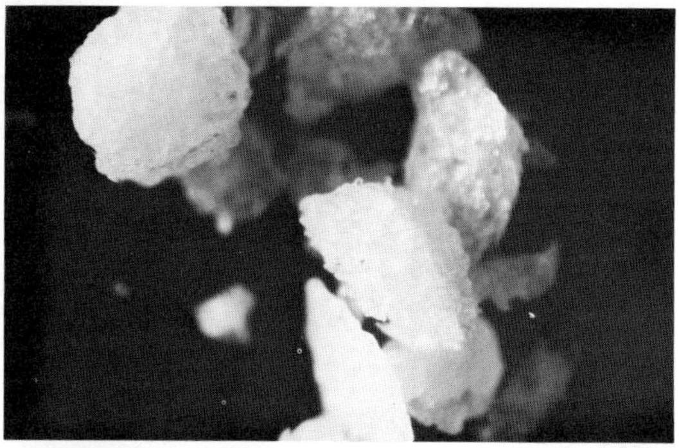

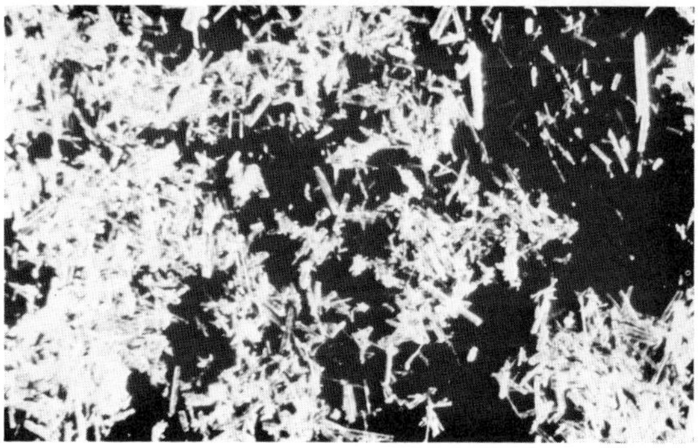

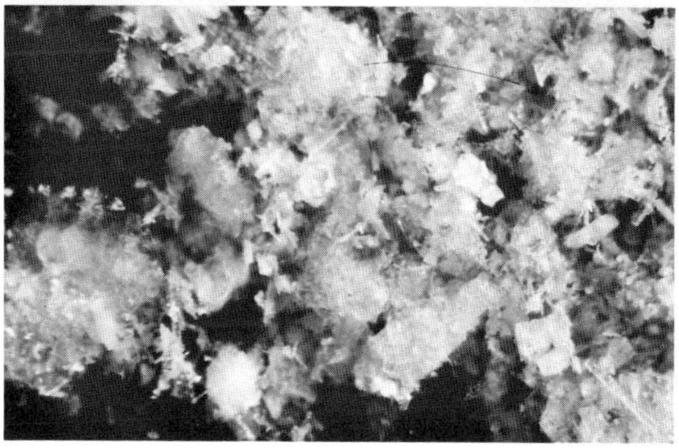

The microphotos shown in these pages were all taken using natural light with a Nikon FM attached to a Nikon microscope. They are reproduced here at approximately 70x. (photos 5-22 by G. Pruitt)

The adulterated samples used in these photos contain 25% of the adulterant screened together with the cocaine, with the exception of photo 20 in which 3 parts cocaine were screened together with one part each of three adulterants resulting in a sample that was 50% cocaine. Photo 22 shows cocaine recrystallized with 25% lidocaine. Microscopic examination is of little value for detecting adulterants, especially if the substances are well screened or recrystallized together. It may, however, be used to detect crudely introduced cuts.

left-to-right, from top:

5. The cocaine shown was refined in the U.S.A. and was used as the standard for this book, with various adulterants added for certain tests. In this microphoto, the mica-like layers of its compressed flake are visible.

6. Merck pharmaceutical cocaine is fluffier since the flat crystals are not pressed together.

7. "Peruvian flake" is less granular, but similar to the standard.

8. "Bolivian rock" is granular, but the translucent crystals are not flat like the "flake."

9. Mannitol, the most common cut, consists of small needlelike crystals.

10. When screened together with cocaine, the mannitol needles are barely visible among the cocaine flakes.

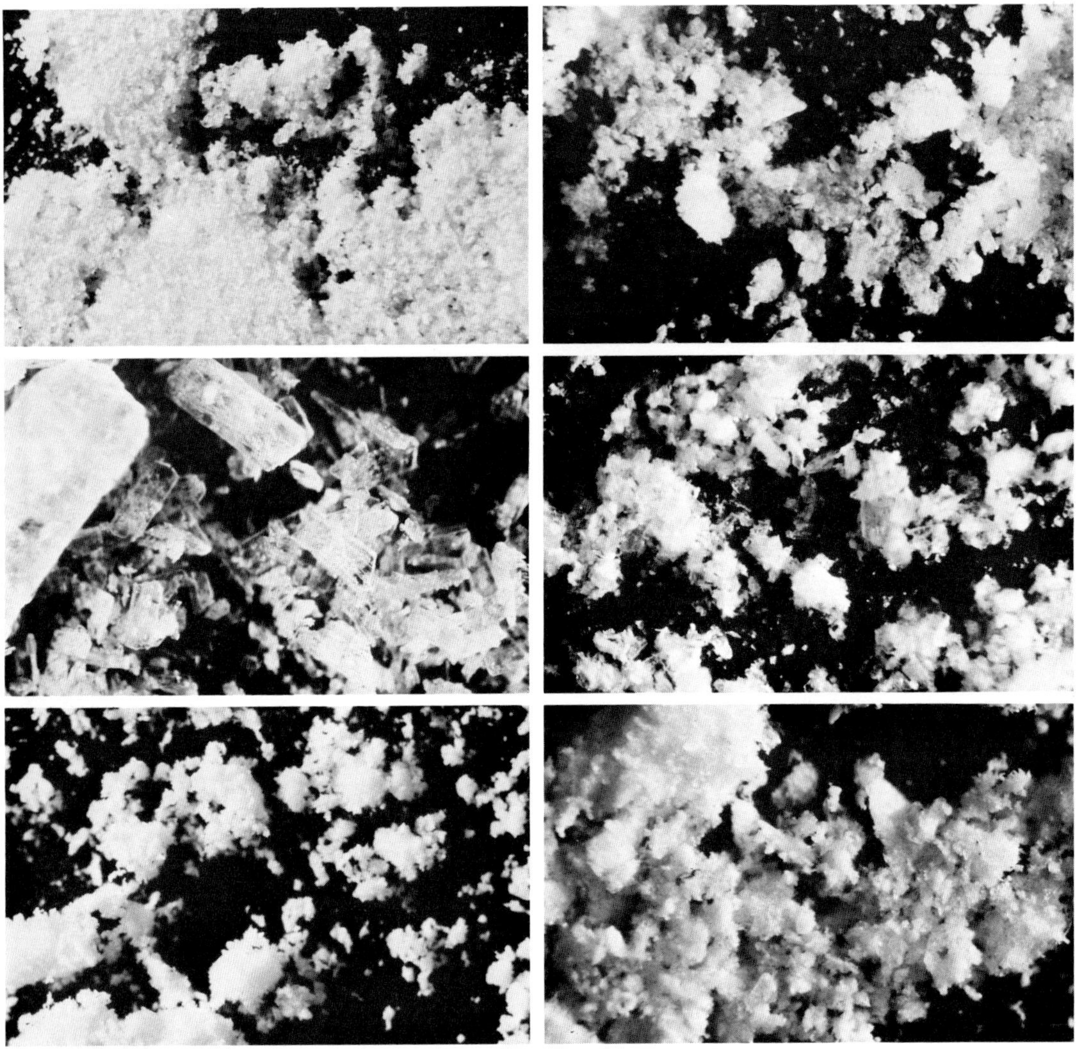

top row:

11. Lactose is an amorphous powder consisting of small uniform particles.

12. When screened with cocaine, lactose particles blend well with the flakes, making detection difficult.

middle row:

13. Inositol consists of rectangular flat crystals of uneven size.

14. When screened with cocaine, the larger crystals of inositol are visible, but the small ones blend in.

bottom row:

15. Caffeine is an amorphous powder consisting of very fine particles.

16. When screened with cocaine, the fine caffeine particles coat the flat surface of the cocaine crystals and dull the appearance.

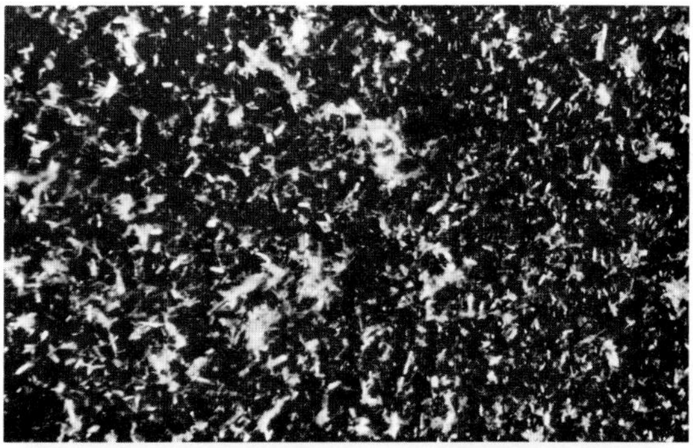
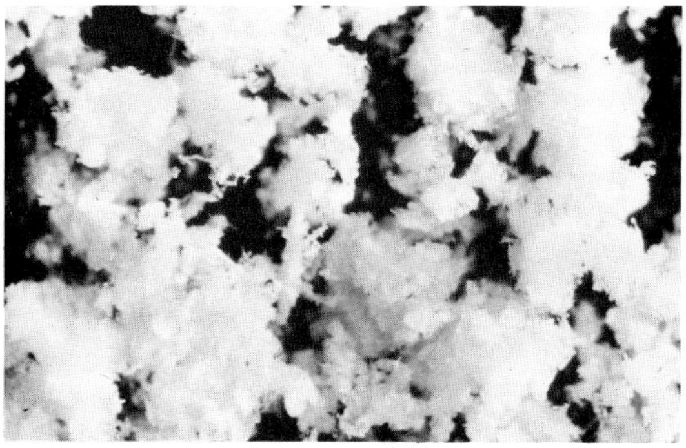
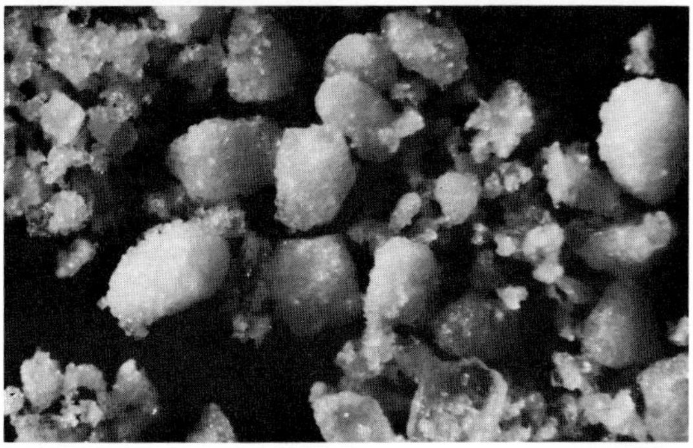
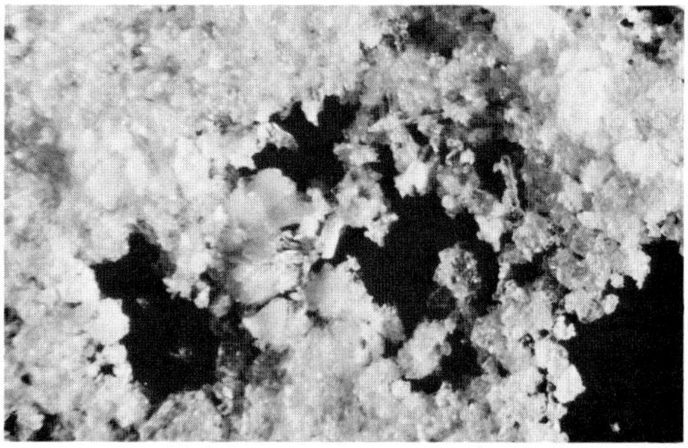
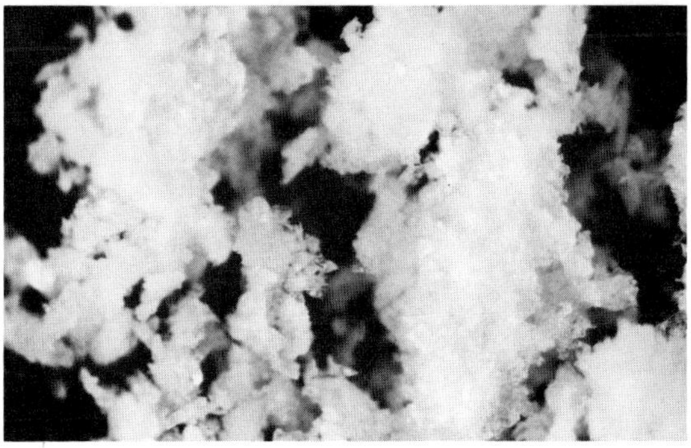
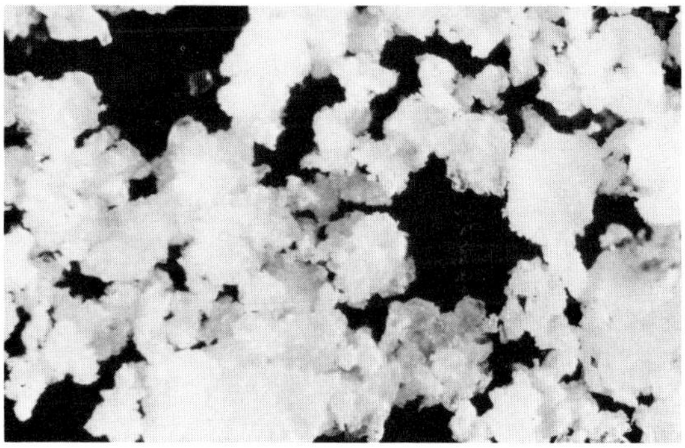

top row:

17. Quinine sulfate consists of small needles and rods.

18. When screened with cocaine, the short hairlike needles of quinine sulfate are visible at the edges of the cocaine flakes.

middle row:

19. Illicit amphetamine, "street speed," resembles "Bolivian rock," but has a duller appearance.

20. Lactose, mannitol, and speed screened together with cocaine are barely detectable. Close examination reveals a few individual mannitol crystals, but the lactose and speed are not distinguishable.

bottom row:

21. A screened mixture of cocaine and lidocaine base cannot be easily distinguished by microscopic examination. However, lidocaine base can be detected with the Clorox or melting point tests.

22. When lidocaine hydrochloride is crystallized with cocaine, as is sometimes done in illicit labs, the resulting product is virtually indistinguishable from cocaine. However, it may be detected with the Clorox test.

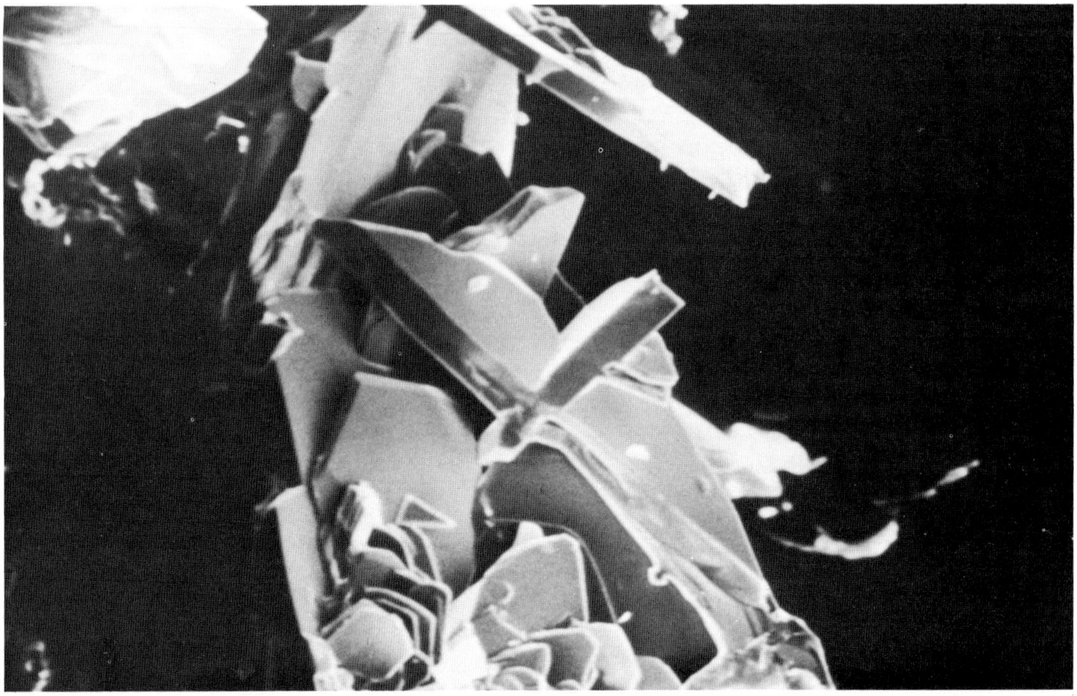

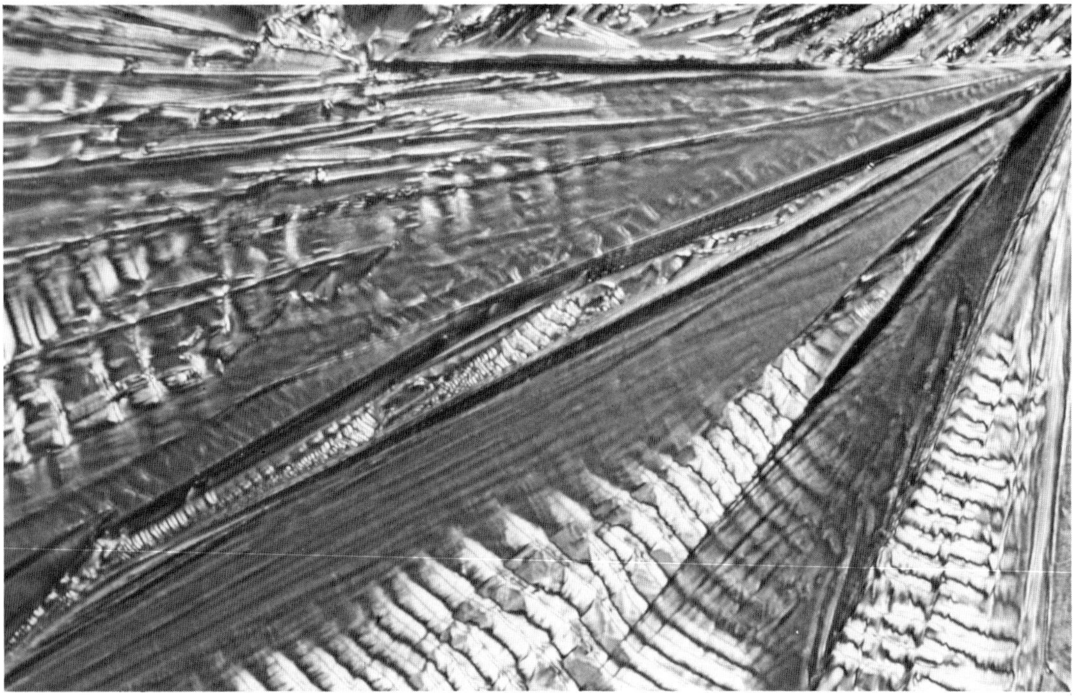

23. This scanning electron micrograph of Merck pharmaceutical cocaine shows the thin, flat crystals. (photos this page: courtesy P. Stamets)

24. The geometric layered structure of a single flake of Merck cocaine is graphically displayed in this micrograph using polarized light.

gram is placed on a coarse screen. Tapping on the side of the screen with a knife or similar device will cause the finer particles (the duff) to pass through while holding back the pieces. The following tests are then done to both samples to see if the pieces and the duff are the same.

Solubility

Cocaine hydrochloride will dissolve in many organic solvents, while many of the substances used as adulterants will not. This principle can be utilized to determine the amount of material which is definitely not cocaine. Since consuming cocaine by nasal inhalation is dependent on its solubility in water, this solvent is the logical place to begin.

A gram of cocaine hydrochloride will dissolve in 0.5 milliliter of distilled water at room temperature. In testing an unknown sample, these proportions are maintained. A small amount (approximately 10 milligrams) of cocaine is placed in a level teaspoon. One drop of very cold water is added so that it will run down to the center of the spoon where the cocaine has been placed. Pure illicit cocaine will dissolve immediately. Anything which does not dissolve is not cocaine hydrochloride.

The same procedure outlined above is used to test the solubility of cocaine in methanol. Cocaine hydrochloride is totally soluble in methanol. Cocaine which has been adulterated with lactose, inositol, quinine, or mannitol will leave traces of undissolved material in the spoon. As with the water test, only one drop of solvent (methanol) is used. A large enough quantity of solvent will dissolve almost anything.

The solubility chart shows how these principles apply to other solvents listed. Water and methanol are the most commonly used, but some testers do use others.

(Continued on page 90)

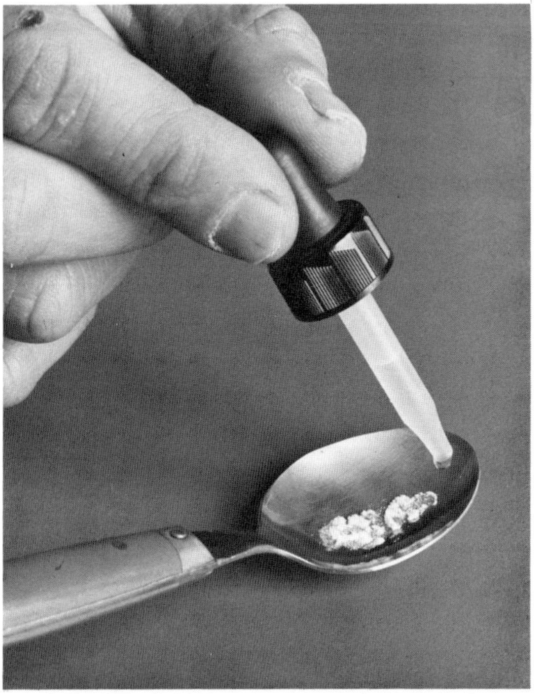

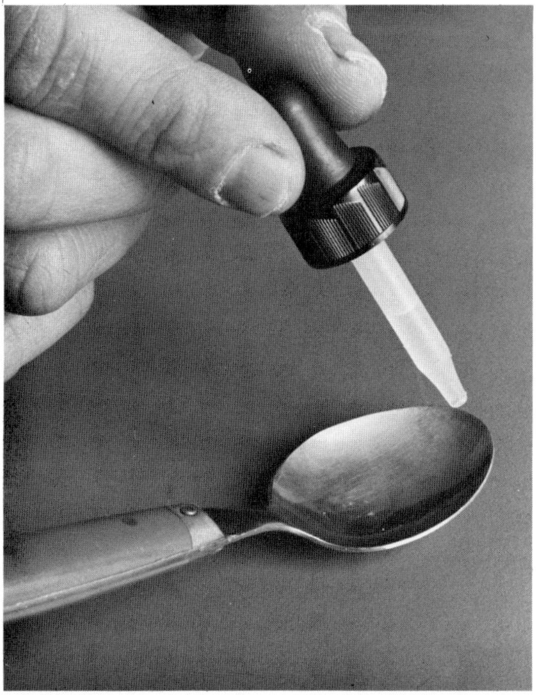

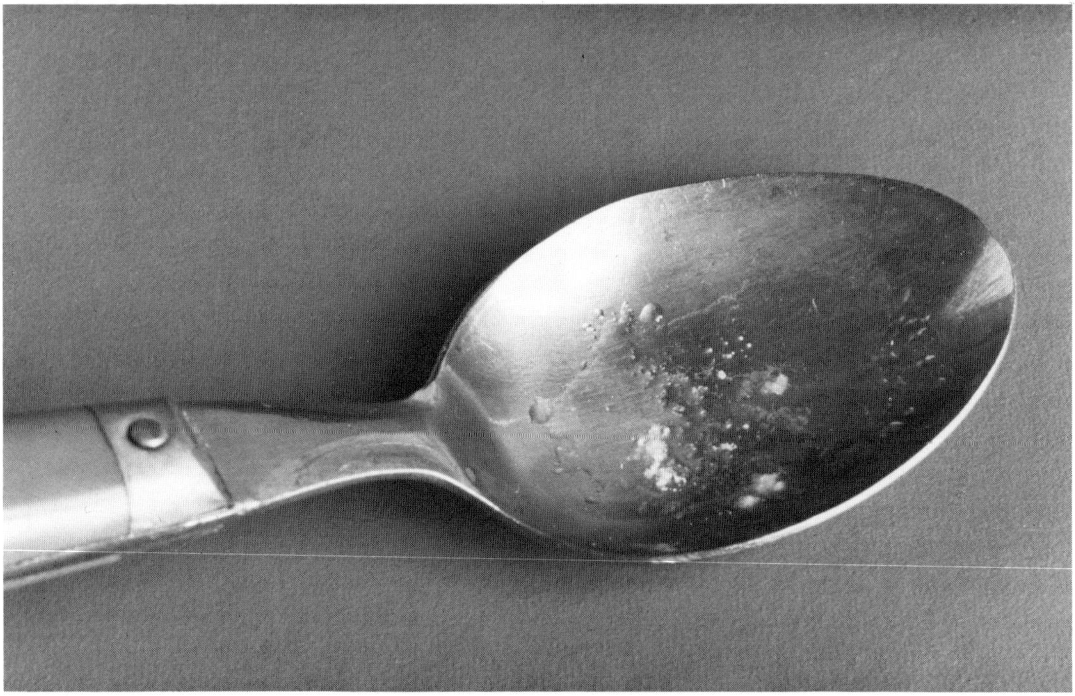

25. When doing the solubility test, a drop of solvent is placed near the edge of the spoon and allowed to run down to the sample.

26. When methanol or water is added to uncut cocaine hydrochloride, the sample dissolves completely within seconds.

27. This sample contains 25% inositol. When methanol is added, much of the cut remains undissolved.

SOLUBILITIES OF COCAINE AND COMMON ADULTERANTS

Acetone=Acet, Chloroform=Chlr, Carbon Disulfide=CD, Benzene=Benz,
Ethyl Acetate=EtAc, soluble=sol, slightly soluble=sl sol, insoluble=insol,
if a number is given it is the amount of solvent needed to dissolve one gram at 25°C

Substance	Water	Diethyl Ether	Petroleum Ether	Methanol	Ethanol	Other
Amphetamine sulfate ("speed")	8.8				515 (95%)	
Benzocaine	sl sol	sol	sol	sol	sol	Chlr-sol
Benzoylecgonine	sol in hot water	insol	insol	sol	sol	
Butacaine base						
Butacaine sulfate	1	insol	insol	v sol in warm	sol in warm	Acet-sol, Chlr-sol
Caffeine	46	530	sl sol	75	66	Acet-50, Chlr-5.5, EtAc-sol
Cocaine base	insol (600)	3.5	30-50	sol	6.5	Acet-5, liquid petrolatum-30-50, Chlr-0.7, oil turpentine-12, olive oil-12, EtAc-sol, CD-sol
Cocaine hydrochloride	0.5	insol	insol	sol	3.2	Acet-insol, Chlr-12.5, oils-insol, glycerol-insol
Cocamine base	insol	sol	sl sol	sol	sol	Acet-sol
Cocamine hydrochloride	sol	insol	insol	sol	sol	Acet-sl sol
Ecgonine base	5	sl sol	sl sol	20	67	Acet-sl sol, Chlr-sl sol, EtAc-75, Benz-sl sol
Ecgonine hydrochloride	sol				sl sol	
Ephedrine base	sol	sol	sol		sol	Chlr-sol, oils-sol
Ephedrine sulfate	1.3	sl sol		90	sol	Chlr-insol
Hygrine base	sl sol	sl sol	sol	sol	sol	Acet-sol, Chlr-sol
Hygrine hydrochloride	sl sol	insol	insol	sol	sol	Acet-sl sol
Inositol	14	insol	insol	sl sol	insol	Acet-sl sol
Lactose	5.0	insol	insol	sl sol	sl sol	Acet-insol, Chlr-insol
Lidocaine base	insol	sol	sol	sol	sol	Chlr-sol, Benz-sol, oils-sol
Lidocaine hydrochloride	sol	insol	insol	sol	sol	Chlr-sol

continued

Some solvents mentioned here and many solvents used routinely in laboratories are toxic and/or flammable (possibly explosive). Working with them where ventilation is inadequate creates a LIFE THREATENING situation. Safe use of such solvents is a complex problem which professional laboratories have solved; any layman using such solvents is risking his life.

Solubilities of Cocaine and Common Adulterants (continued)

Substance	Water	Diethyl Ether	Petroleum Ether	Methanol	Ethanol	Other
Mannitol	5.5	insol	insol	sl sol	83	Pyridine-sol, Aniline-sol Glycerol-18
Pemoline,magnesium	insol	insol				Acet-insol
Phenylpropanolamine base	insol	sol	sol			
Phenylpropanolamine hydrochloride	sol	insol	insol		sol	Chlr-insol, Benz-insol
Procaine base	insol (200)	sol	sol	sol	sol	Chlr-sol, Benz-sol
Procaine hydrochloride	1.0	insol	insol	15	30	Chlr-sl sol
Quinine sulfate	insol (810)	sl sol		sl sol	120	Chlr-sl sol
Sucrose	0.5	insol	insol	100	170	Acet-insol, Chlr-insol, Glyserol-sol, Pyridine-sol
Tetracaine base	insol	sol	sol	sol	sol	Acet-sol
Tetracaine hydrochloride	7	insol	insol	sol	sol	Benz-sol

Clorox II — A Revised Look at the Clorox Test

The idea behind the clorox* test is that adulterants in cocaine behave differently from cocaine when a pinch of the sample is sprinkled on the surface of a glass of laundry bleach. There was no test outlined in the *Cocaine Consumer's Handbook* which received greater attention or was the subject of more controversy than the clorox test. In fact, the publicity it received probably did more to call attention to the need for cocaine testing than any other single factor. History may well remember the clorox test as the major impetus towards cleaning up a very black market.

The increase in public awareness about cocaine brings with it the need for more reliable means of testing. Where-

(Continued on page 100)

* The name "clorox test" has only a historical connection to the brand name. The standard composition of laundry bleach is 5.25% (by weight) sodium hypochlorite and any such solution can be used to do the test. The name "clorox test" became the accepted street term in the late 1960s.

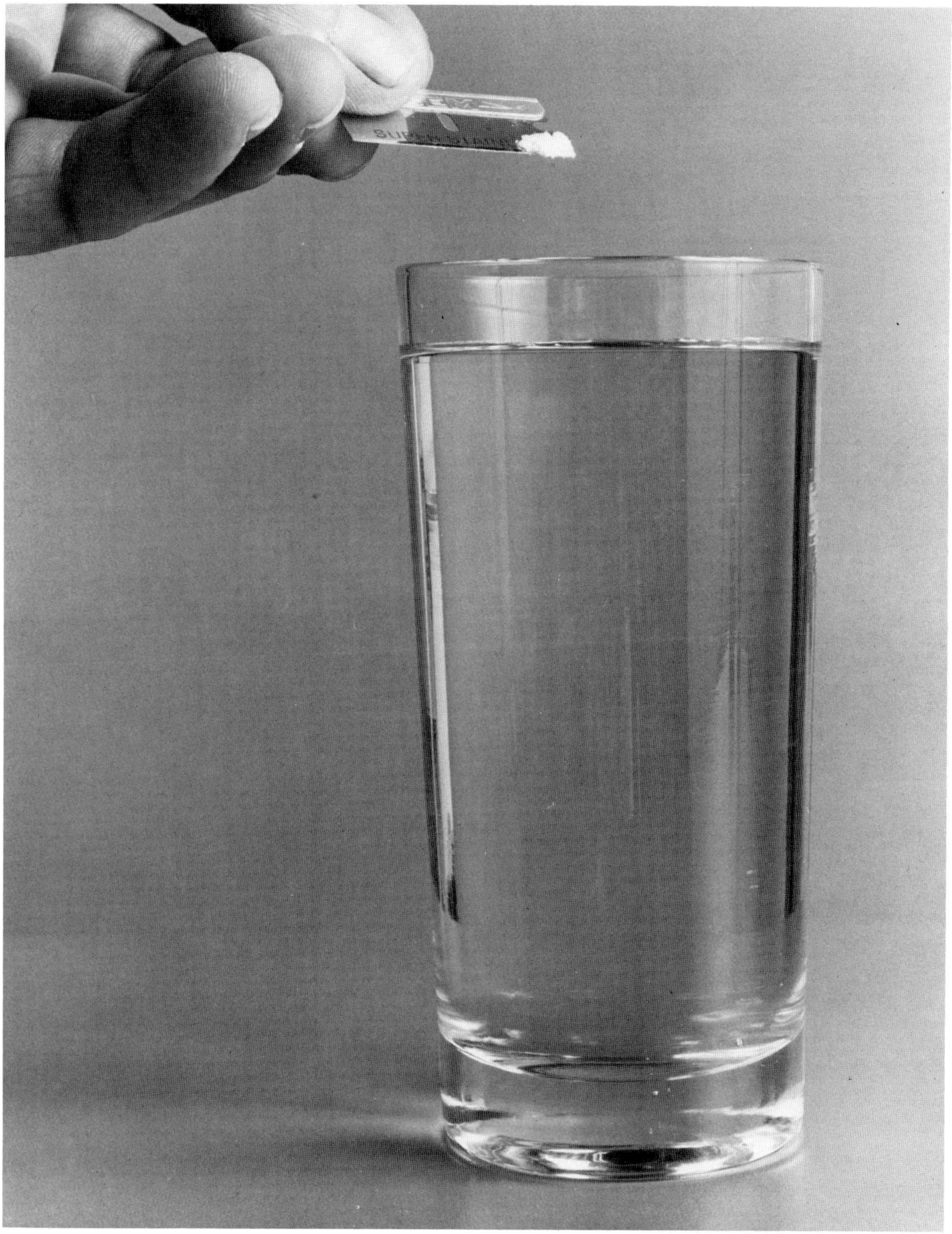

28. When performing the Clorox test, a pinch (about 10 milligrams) of finely chopped sample is dropped into a tall glass of Clorox bleach. Results of the Clorox test are shown in the following pages.

29. Impact

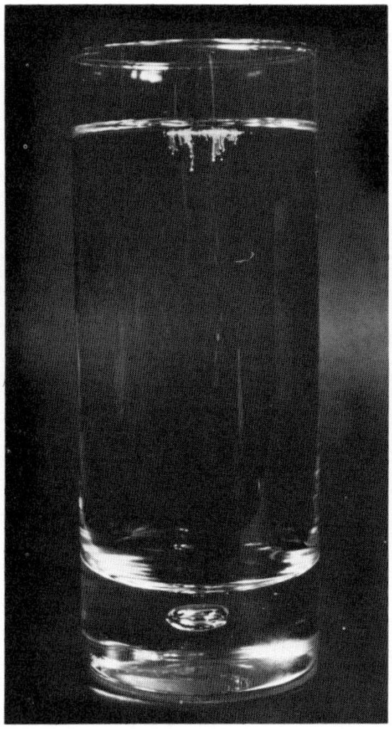

30. 5 sec.

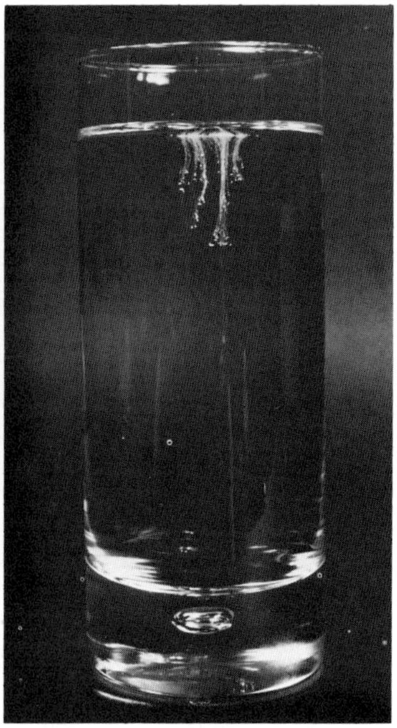

31. 10 sec.

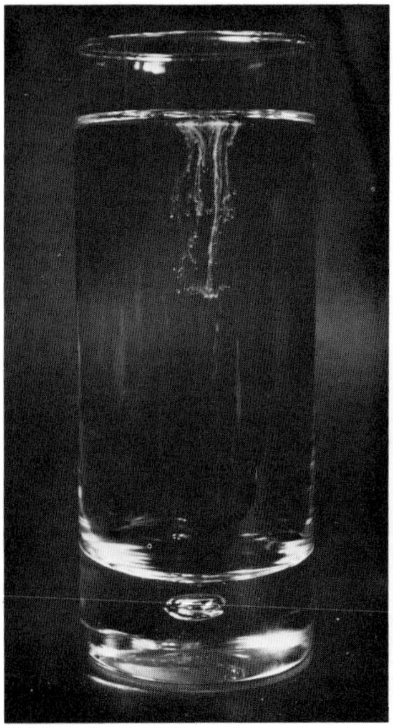

32. 15 sec.

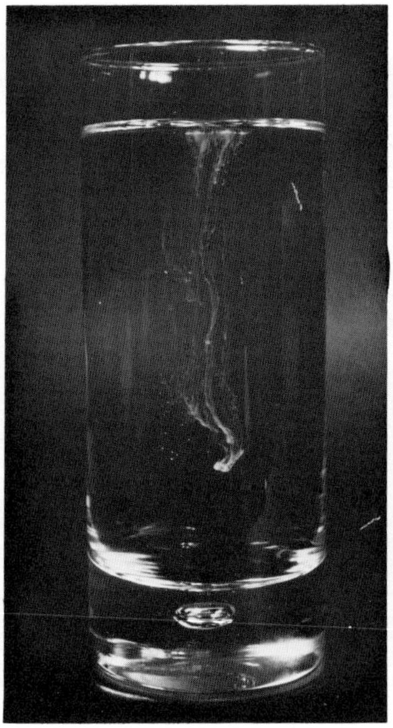

33. 30 sec.

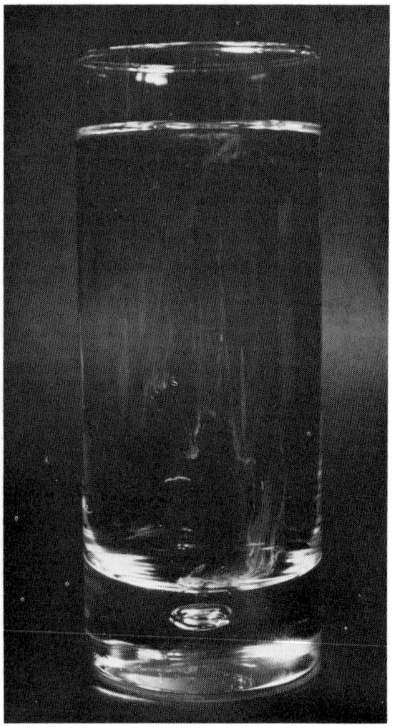

34. 60 sec.

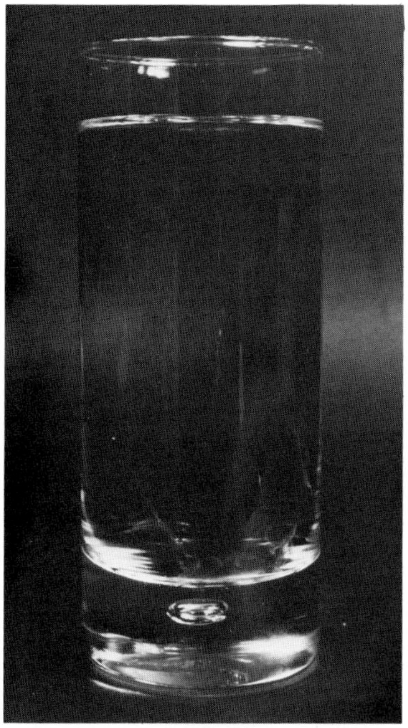

35. 120 sec.

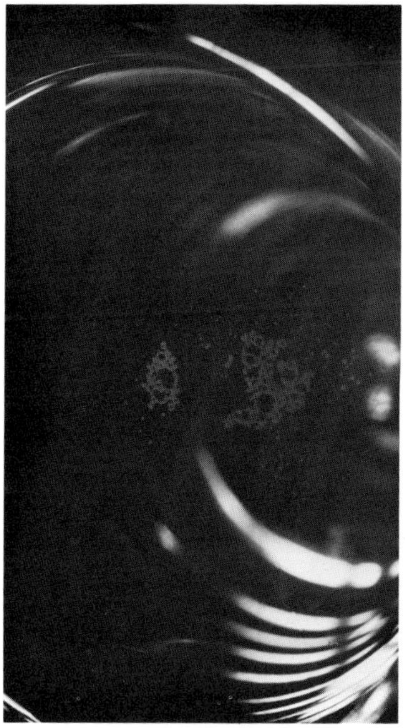

36. Residue

29.-36. These photos show the Clorox test results using about 20 milligrams of highly-refined illicit cocaine ("Book Standard") dropped into a six-inch-tall glass filled with Clorox bleach at room temperature (20°C). The sample hesitates on the surface for a few seconds and then slowly falls in milky trails, leaving no residue on the bottom and only a small oily residue on top.

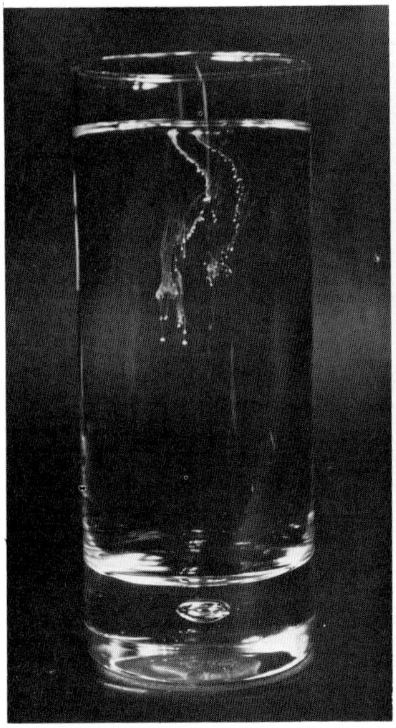

37. 15 sec.

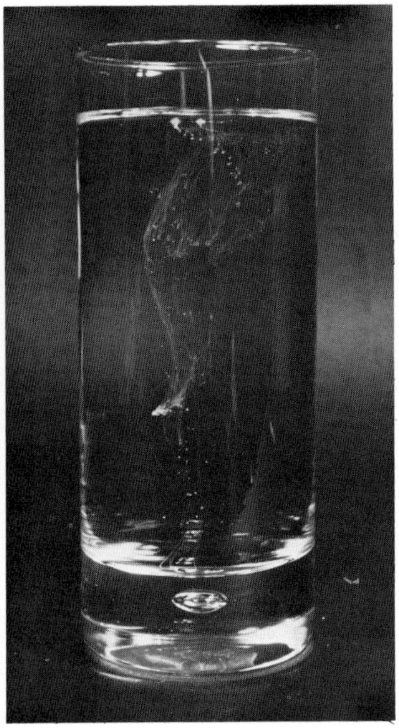

38. 30 sec.

37.&38. Merck pharmaceutical cocaine reacts much the same way as the refined illicit cocaine, as shown in these photos at left, taken 15 and 30 seconds after impact.

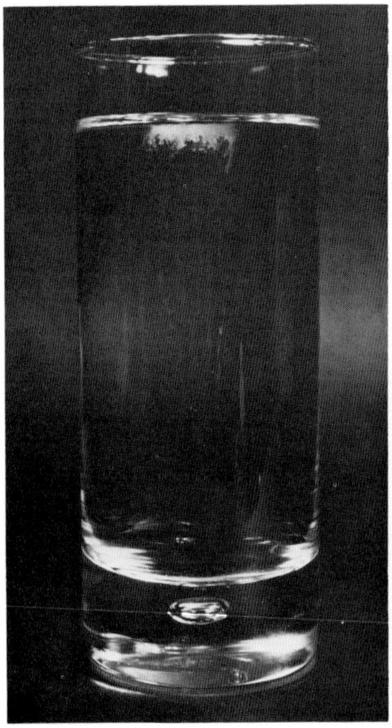

39. 15 sec.

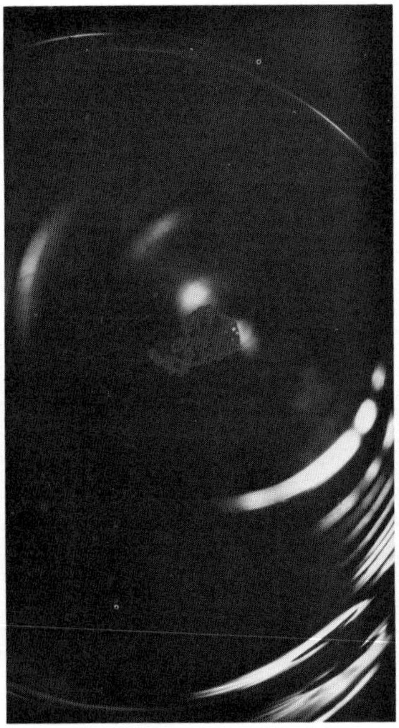

40. Residue

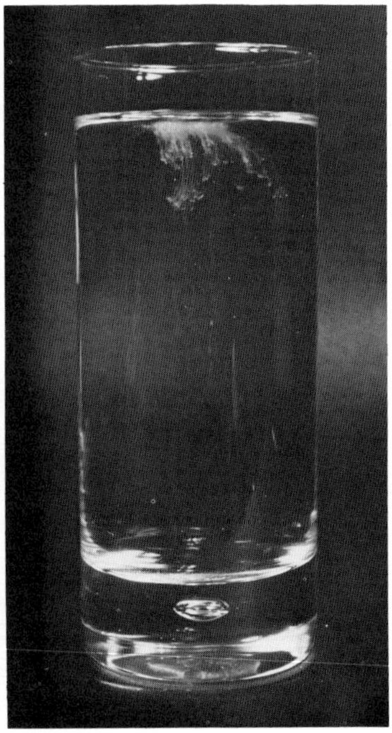

41. 30 sec.

39.&40. The Peruvian style flake refined in the U.S.A. hesitates longer on the surface due to the presence of a higher percentage of oily impurities, as evidenced by the larger residue remaining on the surface.

41. The imported "Bolivian rock" also hesitates due to impurities as shown at 30 seconds after impact.

42.&43. A mixture of 25% mannitol and 75% cocaine hydrochloride (at right) reacts much like the standard. The trails hit the bottom, but eventually disappear.

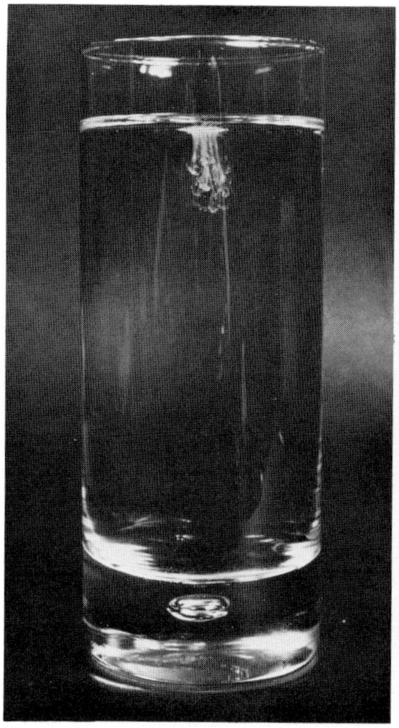

42. 15 sec.

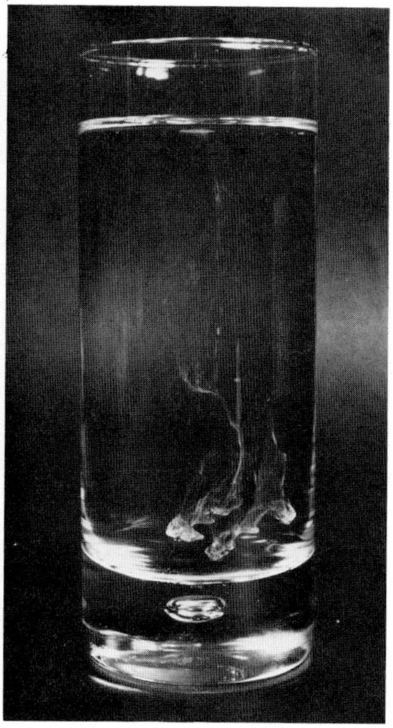

43. 60 sec.

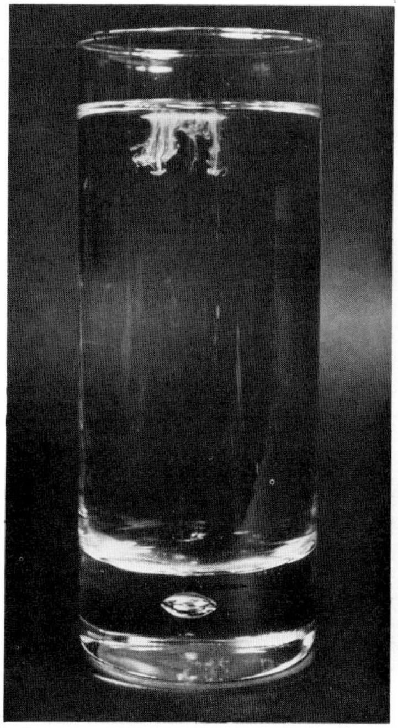

44. 15 sec.

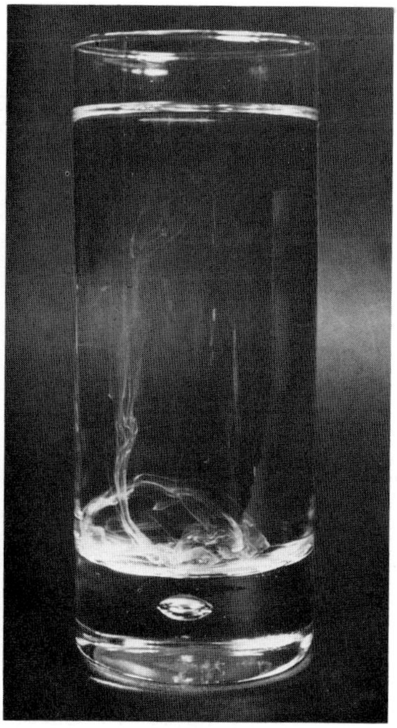

45. 60 sec.

44.&45. A sample with 25% lactose is virtually indistinguishable from the standard after 15 seconds, but after 60 seconds the trails on the bottom are still pronounced.

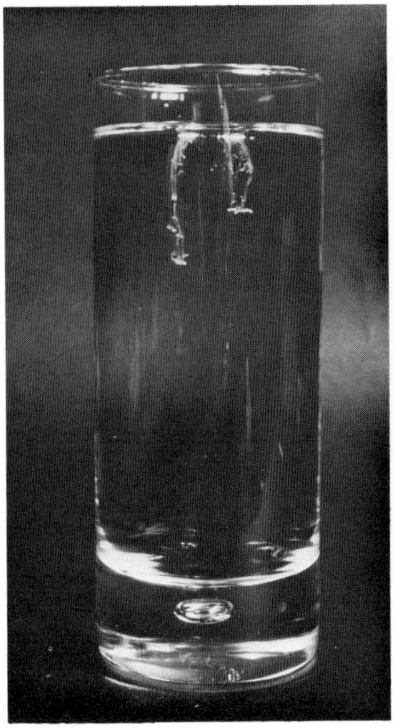

46. 15 sec.

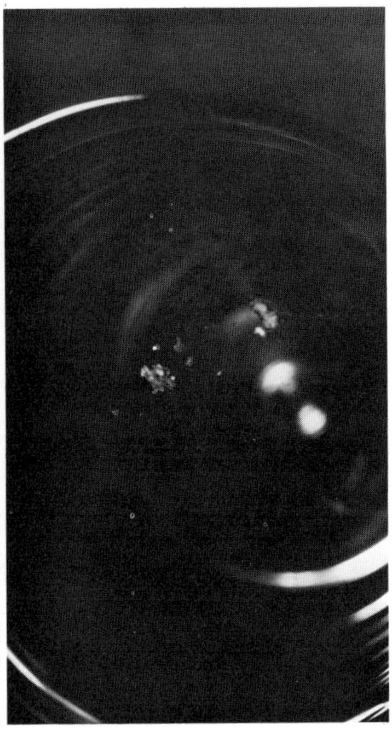

47. Residue

46.&47. A sample with 25% quinine falls with fewer trails than the standard, and leaves a pink residue on the surface.

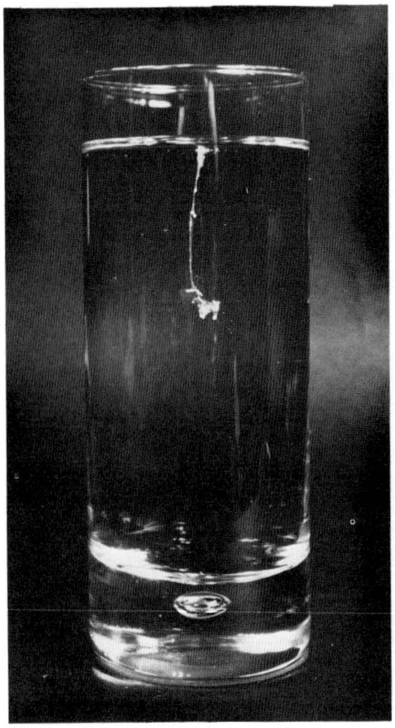

48. 5 sec.

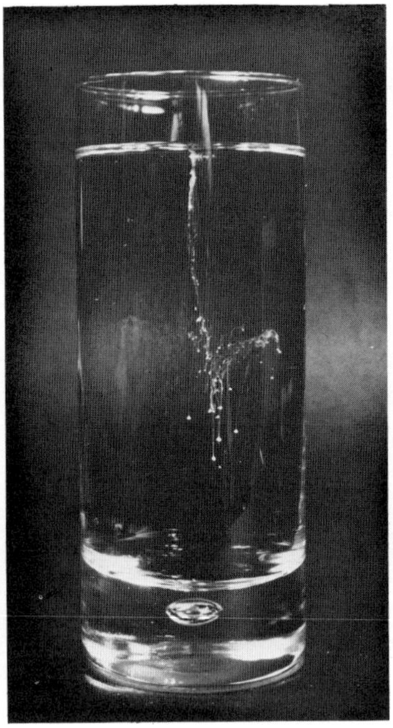

49. 10 sec.

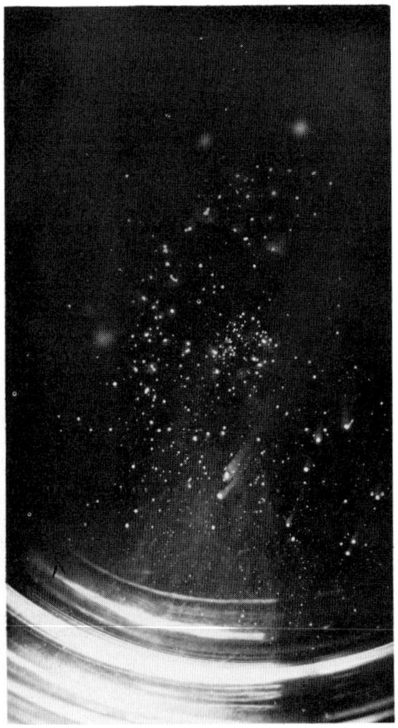

50. Residue

48.,49.,&50. A sample with 25% inositol falls rapidly; the particles of inositol separate from the cocaine and leave a residue on the bottom.

51.&52. A sample with 50% cocaine and the rest a mixture of mannitol, lactose, and speed is barely distinguishable from the standard. However, this mixture fails the foil burn test (see color plate 68 on p.144).

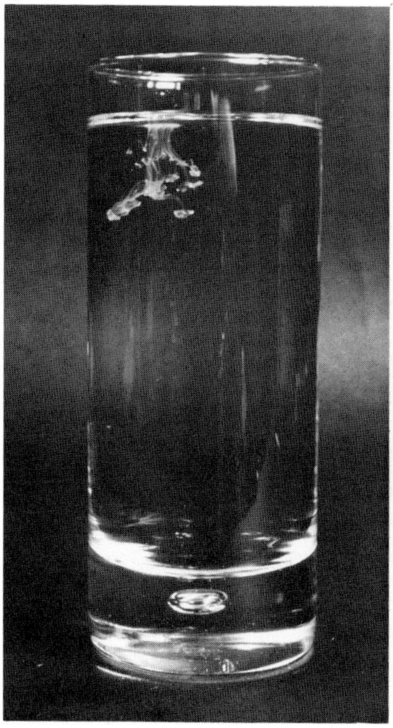

51. 15 sec.

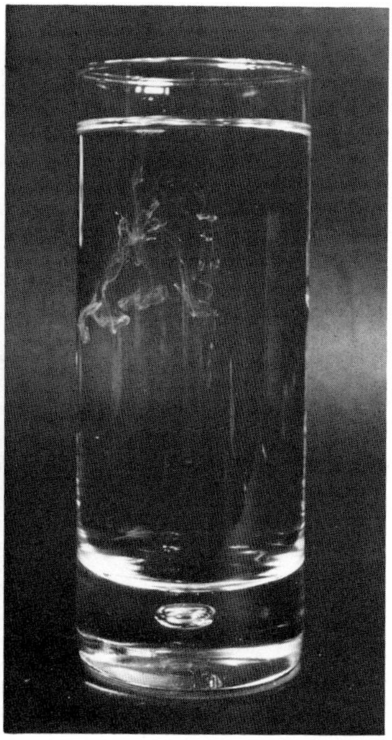

52. 30 sec.

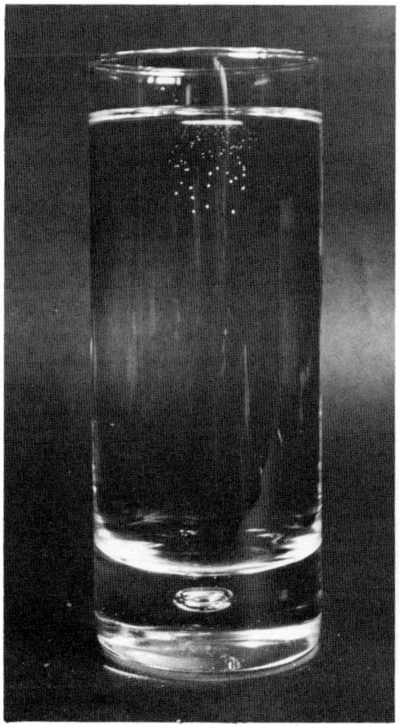

53. 5 sec.

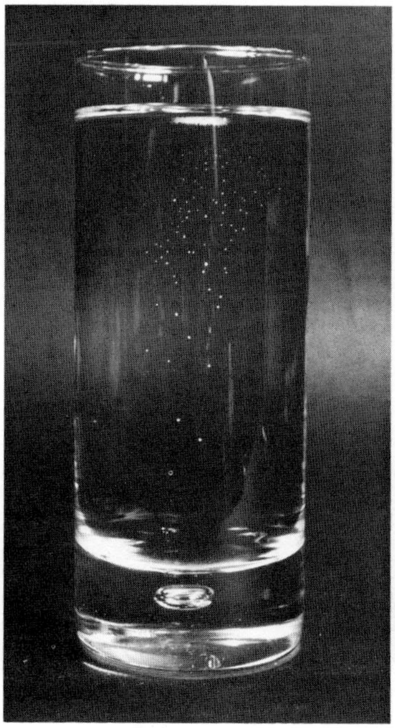

54. 15 sec.

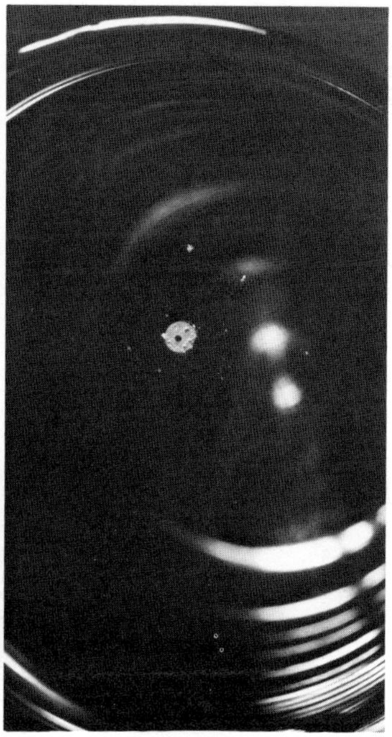

55. Residue

53.,54.,&55. A sample with 25% caffeine separates more quickly than inositol. The cocaine hesitates longer before trailing. The caffeine separates and a distinct white residue forms on top. No residue remains on the bottom.

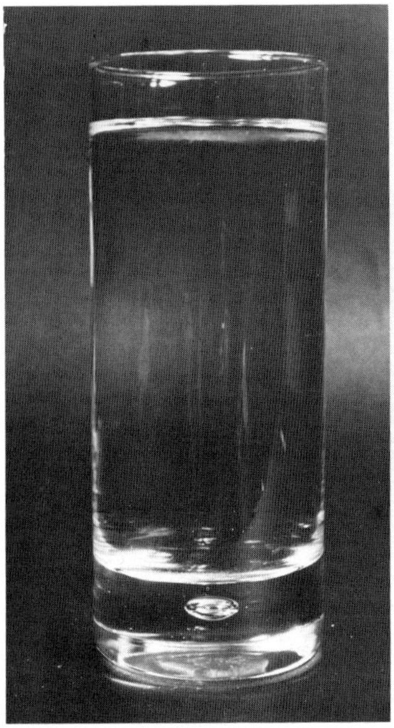

56. 60 sec.

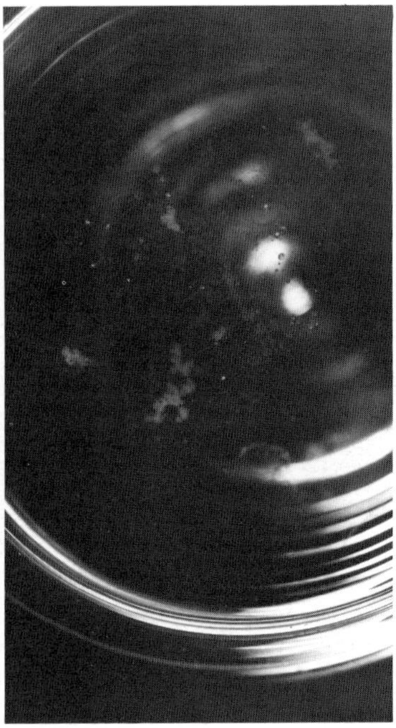

57. Residue

56.&57. A sample with 25% lidocaine base has still not fallen after 60 seconds. After two minutes, a residue remains on the surface.

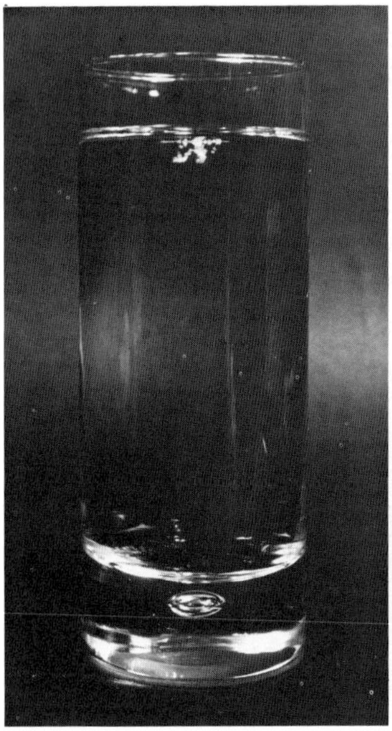

58. Impact

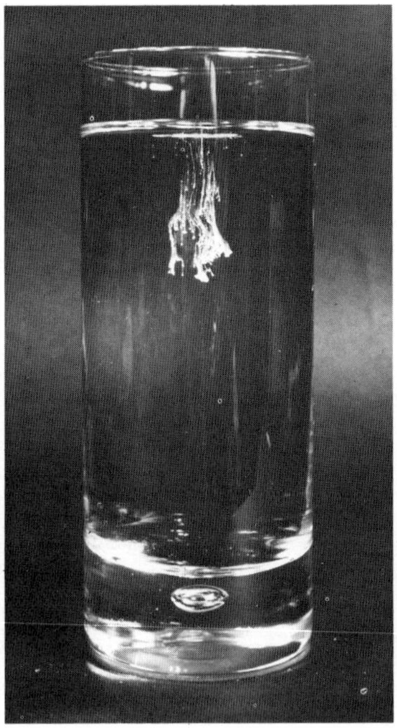

59. 5 sec.

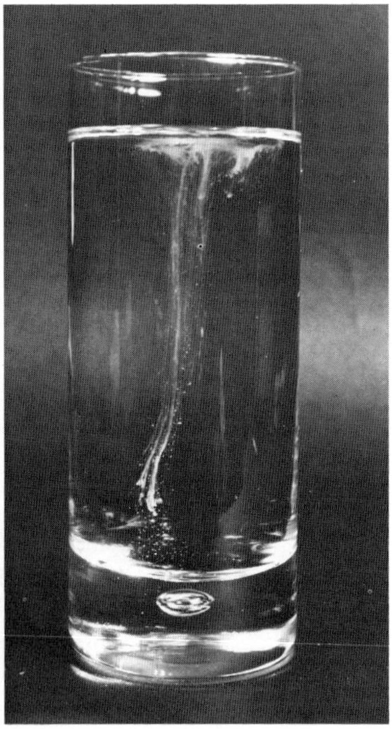

60. 30 sec.

58., 59., &60. A sample with 25% lidocaine begins to fall upon impact. After 5 seconds the trails have fallen substantially further than the standard. At 30 seconds it is still milky on top even though trails are already hitting the bottom.

61.&62. A sample which was analyzed by Pharm Chem as containing only lidocaine and lactose, but not cocaine, did not form trails, danced on the surface, and left an orange residue.

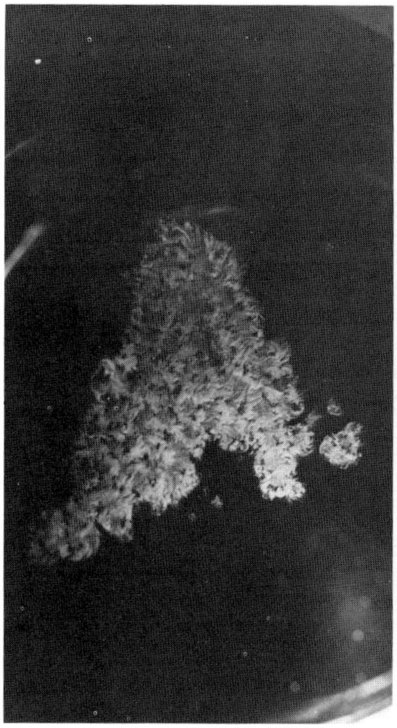

61. Surface

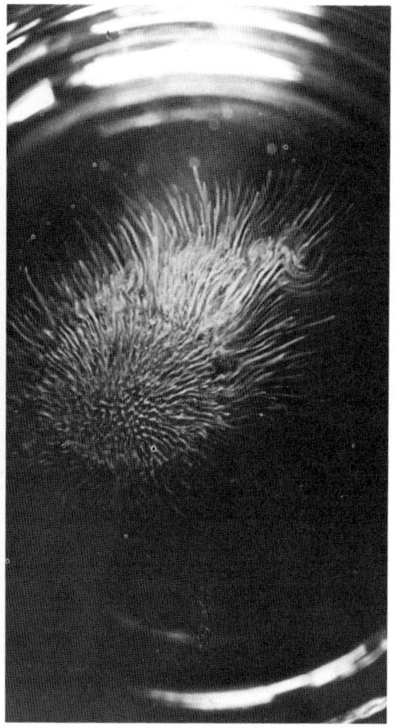

62. Surface

SUMMARY

In summary, the Clorox test is highly subjective. Different testers can look at the same test and come to different conclusions. Caffeine and lidocaine base are the most distinguishable with lidocaine hydrochloride and inositol trailing close behind. Again, the results of several tests considered together can be more conclusive than the Clorox test alone.

as, in 1976, the clorox test could give the consumer a reasonable idea of the quality of an unknown sample of street cocaine, in 1980 the same test cannot even guarantee that cocaine is present. One must understand that in a progressive market like cocaine, dealer awareness keeps pace with consumer awareness. If the consumer finds a new test, the dealer must use a cut which will fool the test. The clorox test may be very effective in detecting a cut which is just mixed in as a powder but ineffective if the same cut is introduced in some step of making the cocaine hydrochloride.

The nature of illicit cocaine has changed in the past 5 years. Illicit cocaine is seldom refined to the extent that it once was. The additional weight created by the lack of refinement has in some cases replaced adulteration. At least at the source, it is more common for larger shipments of cocaine to be uncut — but unrefined also. It is this lack of refinement which often fools the clorox test. The hygrine oil which has become a component part of illicit cocaine will cause the sample dropped in clorox to hesitate on the surface even longer than would pure cocaine. The result is an excellent looking clorox test which may not reflect the true quality of the cocaine.

Although the reliability of the clorox test has diminished for these reasons, there is still a lot of street cocaine which contains the same sugars and/or local anesthetics which are so plainly visible in clorox. If for this reason alone, the clorox test is still well worth the time for the majority of consumers.*

To perform the clorox test, a tall clear glass is filled with fresh clorox which is at room temperature. The bleach is allowed to stand until the liquid is motionless. A clean knife or razor blade is used to drop a small sample of the cocaine on the top of the clorox. The results are observed.

---

* For example a commercial product (TOOT, the Heavenly Incense) is being used by many as a cocaine substitute and will probably appear as a cut. When TOOT is dropped on bleach it remains on the surface and turns pink; with time, the color darkens to orange and then red. According to Pharm Chem, TOOT contains benzocaine, caffeine, and phenylpropanolamine.

The Foil Burn Test

This simple test is based on the principle that substances which are heated on aluminum foil with a butane lighter will vary in the way that they burn and in the kind of residue which they leave behind. While it will be extremely difficult to establish the identity of the substance or the amount of it which is present, it is easy to determine the differences between cocaine and lactose. Sugar adulterants, like lactose, leave a very dark residue, and doing the foil burn test with a pinch of ordinary sugar can serve as example of sugar adulterants.

At Home

As testing procedures increase in complexity, it becomes more and more difficult for them to be performed on location. There is not only more equipment to transport and set up, but the consumer is also likely to meet with even greater resistance from the seller. For these and other reasons, the melt point test and the cocaine base test are usually done at home, after the purchase has been made.

Although there may be no recourse should either of these tests prove the cocaine to be of inferior quality, there is still value in doing the tests. The experience gained by personally seeing the tests provides information which is helpful in relating the results of the more complicated tests to those of the simpler, on-location tests. Ingesting inferior quality cocaine is a bad practice even if it's free, and with some experience in testing a more informed decision is possible.

The Melting Point Test

The purpose of the melting point test is to identify an unknown substance and determine its purity. This is accomplished by heating the material and noting both the temperature at which it begins to change from a solid to a liquid, and the temperature which is reached at the time that the change is complete. These figures are then compared to those of known substances. Since the melting point of a solid is easily determined and requires minimal

(Continued on page 104)

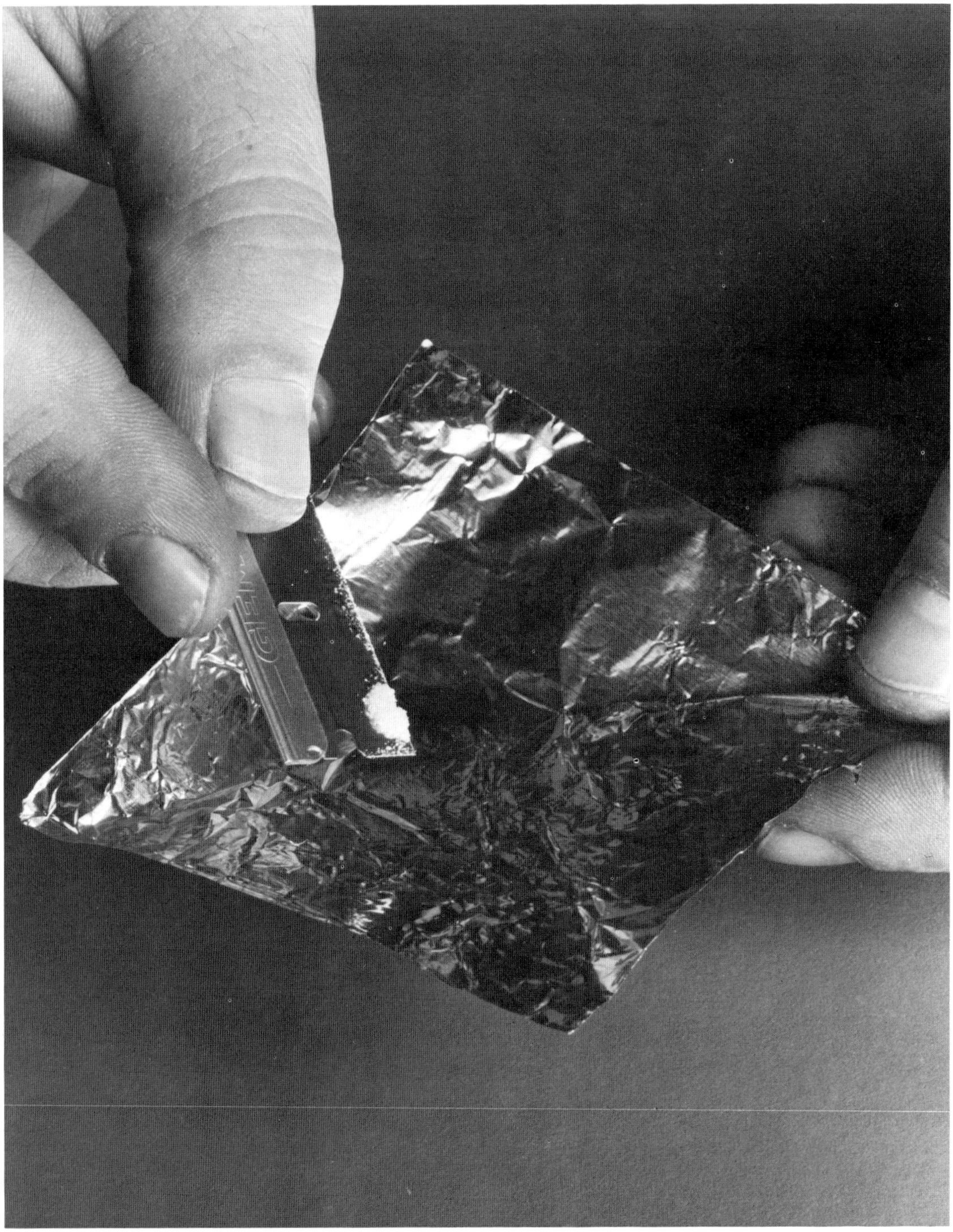

63. A pinch of the sample (about 10 milligrams) is placed on the aluminum foil.

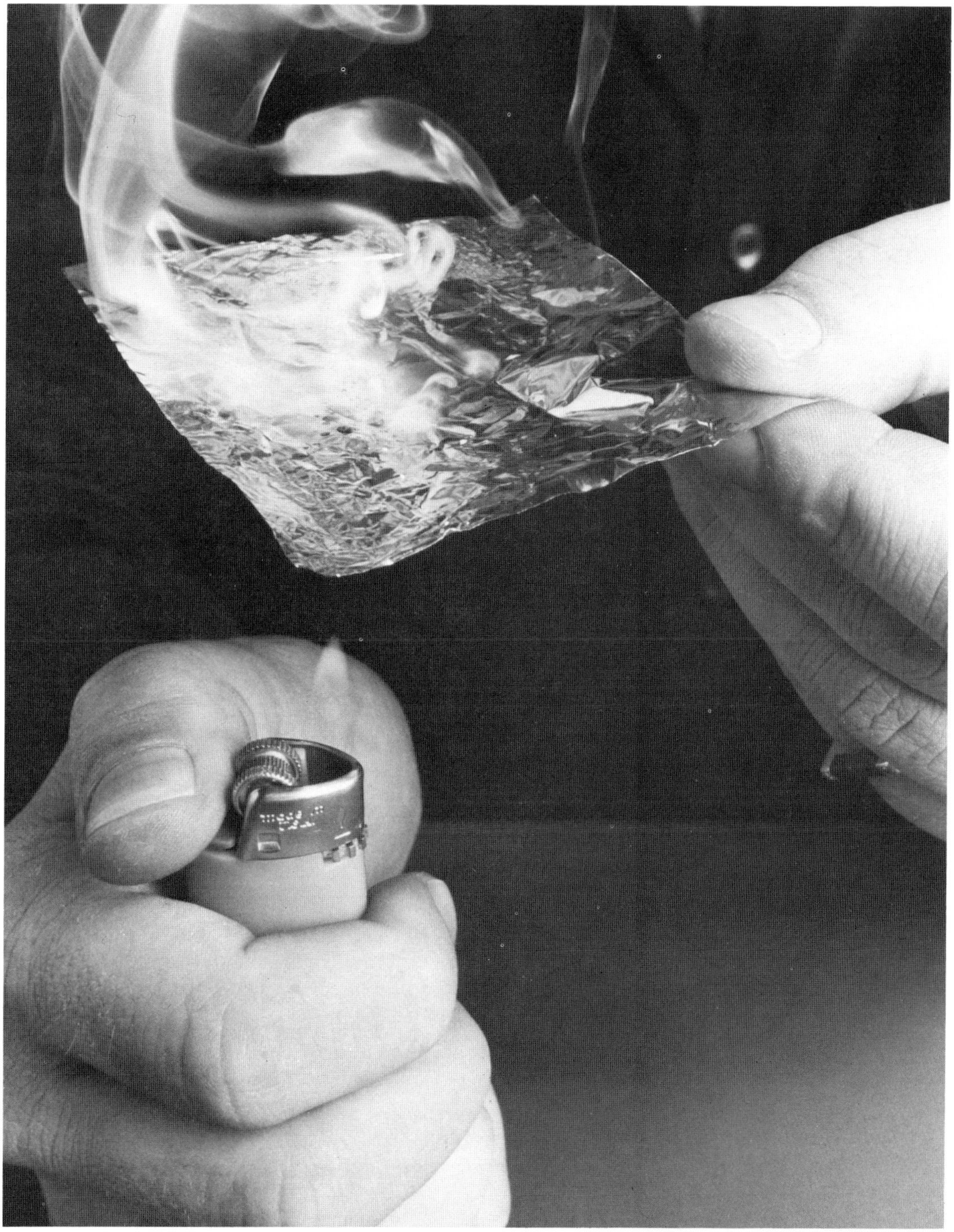

64. The sample is heated very gently from below with a butane lighter. The residue is then examined: for results of various samples, see color photos on p. 144.

use of cocaine, it is the criterion most often used for estimation of purity.

Unlike the boiling point of a liquid, the melting point of a solid is unaffected by changes in barometric pressure. It will, however, be affected by the moisture content of the cocaine, the degree to which it has been refined, impurities and adulterants which are present, and the technical skills and objectivity of the person performing the test. The simplest way to determine the melting point of a solid like cocaine is to observe a sample in a glass capillary tube as it is slowly heated. The first step is to load a dry, finely chopped sample into the open end of a thin-walled capillary tube. The capillary is repeatedly dropped through a straw with the closed end down in order to minimize air pockets while tightly packing the cocaine. The capillary is then attached to a thermometer with the bottom of the closed end of the capillary even with the bottom of the thermometer. The two may then be suspended in an oil bath which can be heated evenly and slowly.

If the melting point of a substance is known, the temperature may be raised rapidly until just before the melting temperature is reached; then, the rate of temperature increase is slowed down to one degree per minute. Since the melting point of illicit cocaine is so varied, the temperature is raised by 10 degrees a minute until the oil is 160°C. The rate of increase is then slowed down to one degree per minute until the melt is complete. If any melting takes place below 160°C., the test is repeated with the rate of increase slowed down before any melting has begun.

Pharmaceutical cocaine hydrochloride, which has no other alkaloids, will melt between 195–197°C. There will be no capillary reaction below 190°C.

Uncut illicit cocaine hydrochloride (made from leaves of *E. coca*) will melt between 187–192°C. The presence of minute impurities may lower the temperature by a few degrees, but there should be no melting below 185°C.

Uncut Potpourri cocaine hydrochloride (made from leaves of varied origin) often has several other alkaloids present with melting points around 180°C. The melt will vary from 182–186°C., depending on the amount of other alkaloids which are present. There should not be any reaction below 180°C.

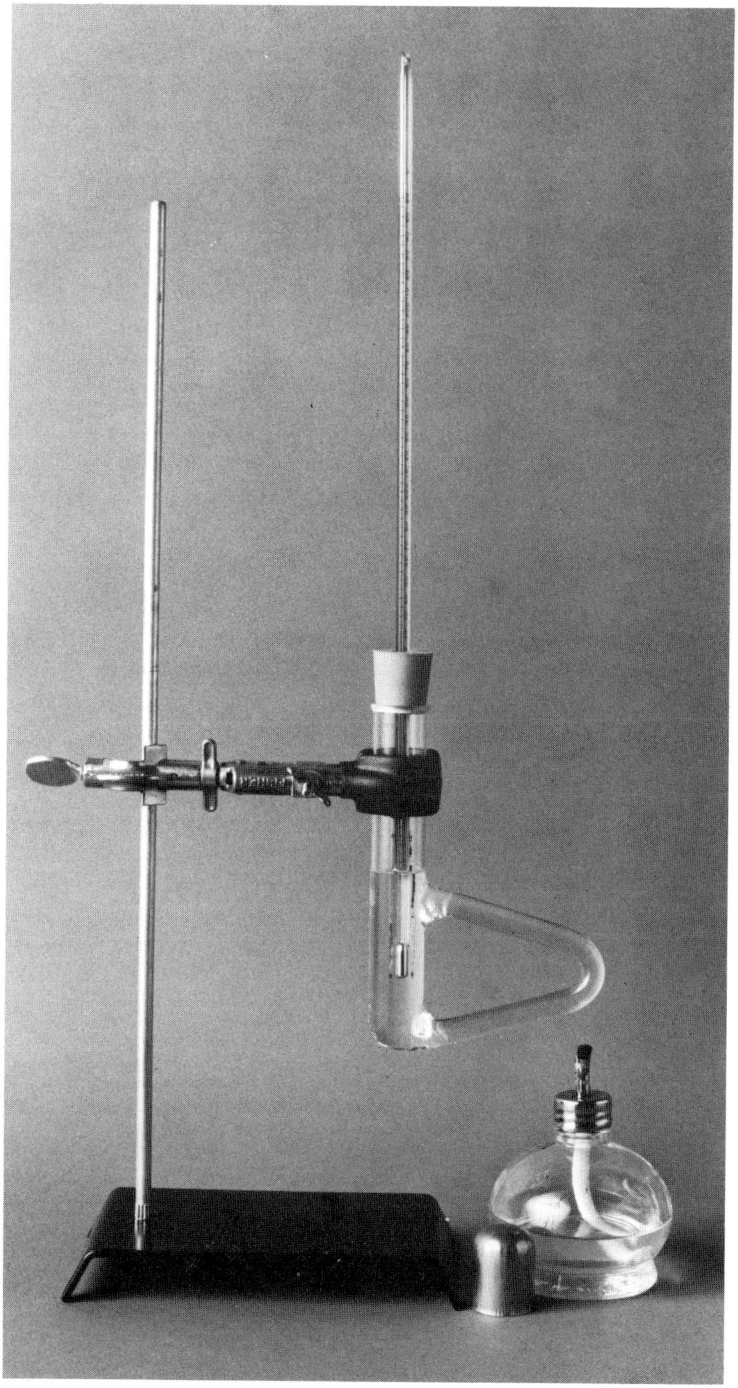

65. The classical set-up and equipment for performing the melting point test: capillaries, a lab thermometer, a lab stand, and a Thiele-Dennis tube filled with mineral oil heated by an alcohol burner.

Very few consumers will be able to obtain cocaine which will melt in this way. The majority of uncut illicit cocaine will have impurities that will lower the melting point to approximately 180°C. The lower melting point and wider spread (three to five degrees) usually occurs with cocaine which has some discoloration, a distinguishable odor, and an oily consistency. A similar melting point with cocaine which does not have these physical characteristics is usually indicative of adulteration. Often, a cut is added in such a way as to indicate superficially that only one substance is present. The absence of odor or discoloration is the tip-off that the lower melting temperature and wider spread has been caused by something other than lack of refinement.

Although many commercial melting point kits have been developed specifically for testing cocaine, none are more accurate than the simple capillary, oil bath system. The needed equipment can be purchased at any scientific supply company and includes the following items:

1. 250° C. thermometer, 360 mm in length
2. Asbestos-sleeved burette clamp, with round jaws, medium size
3. Capillary tubes, one end closed, inside diameter, 0.9–1.1 mm, length 90 mm
4. Alcohol burner and alcohol
5. Melting point tube (Thiele)
6. Rubber stopper
7. Mineral oil
8. Several small, thick rubber bands
9. Laboratory stand (optional)

Many people will prefer the ease of operation offered by the commercial electric melt systems. The systems which are accurate enough for meaningful tests all have the following features:

1. The thermometer is readable at temperatures between 60°C. and 200°C.
2. The thermometer and sample are in close enough proximity to each other to guarantee that they are at the same temperature.

3. The rate of temperature increase is adjustable, the finer the control, the better.
4. Two samples can be tested at the same time.
5. The thermometer is replaceable.
6. The view of the thermometer and sample is not obscured. A magnified view is preferable.

(Continued on page 110)

MELTING POINTS OF COCAINE AND COMMON ADULTERANTS

SUBSTANCE	MELTING POINT °C
Amphetamine sulfate ("speed")	>300
Benzocaine	88-92
Benzoylecgonine	86-92 dec 155 dry
Butacaine base	178-182 bp (boiling point)
Butacaine sulfate	138.5-139.5
Caffeine	238
Cocaine base (pharmaceutical)	98
Cocaine base (illicit)	89-95 (varies with purity)
Cocaine hydrochloride (pharmaceutical)	195
Cocaine hydrochloride (illicit)	187-192 (varies with purity)
Cocamine base	80 (approx.)
Cocamine hydrochloride	175-180 (approx.)
Ecgonine base	198
Ecgonine hydrochloride	246
Ephedrine base	79
Ephedrine sulfate	247
Hygrine base	193-195 (boiling point)
Hygrine hydrochloride	
Inositol	225-227
Lactose	201-202
Lidocaine base	68-69
Lidocaine hydrochloride	127-129
Mannitol	166-168
Pemoline, magnesium	259
Phenylpropanolamine base	101-101.5
Phenylpropanolamine hydrochloride	190-194
Procaine base	61
Procaine hydrochloride	153-156
Quinine sulfate	238
Sucrose	decomposes 160-186
Tetracaine base	
Tetracaine hydrochloride	147-150

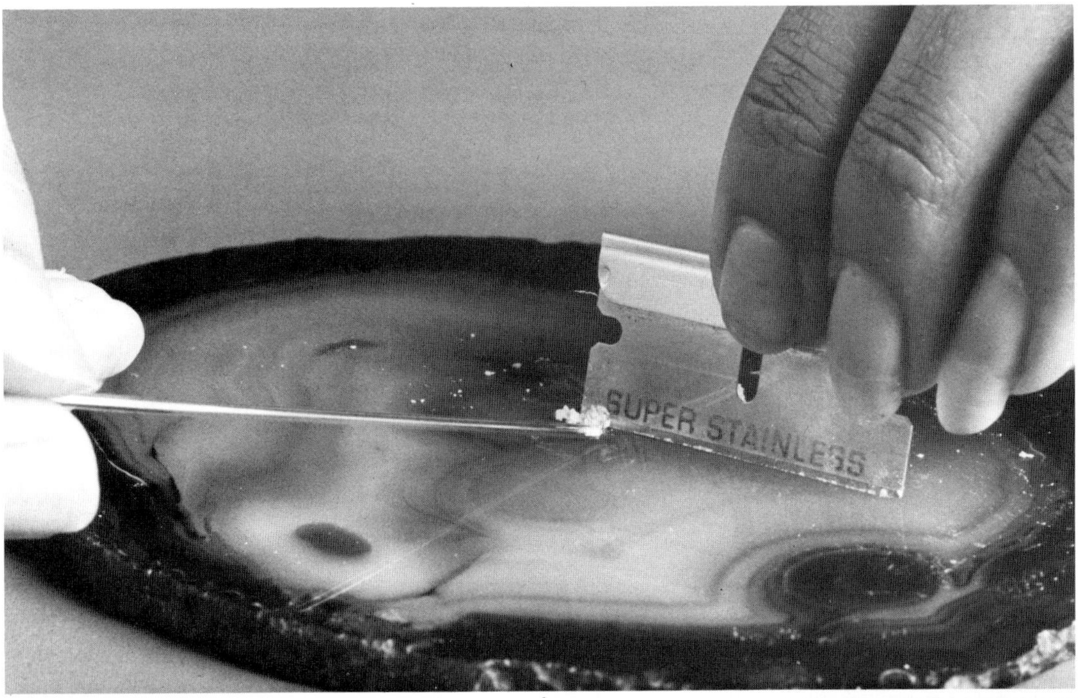

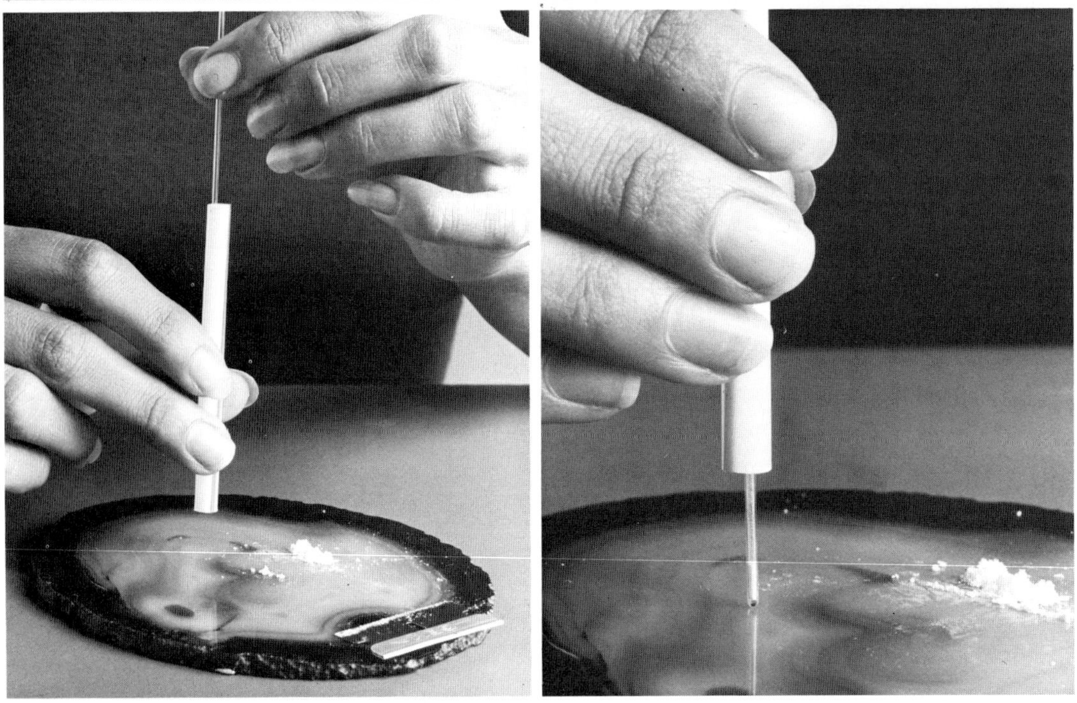

66. A razor blade is used to load the capillary with finely chopped dried sample.

67.&68. The capillary is repeatedly dropped through a straw to pack the sample to the bottom and minimize air pockets.

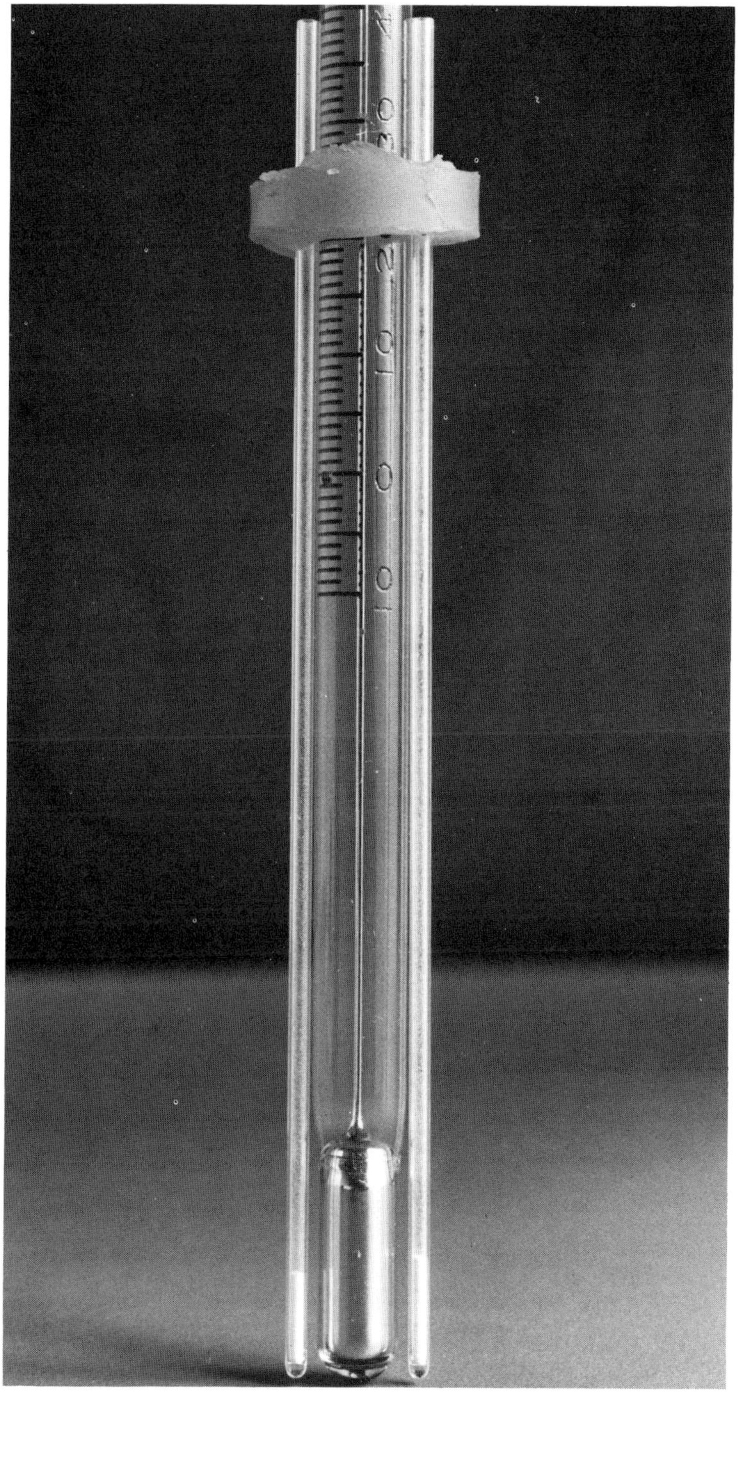

69. The capillaries are attached so the samples are next to the thermometer bulb. (Results of the melting point test are shown in color plates on pp. 142-143.)

The Cocaine Base Test

The purpose of the cocaine base test is to give the consumer a reliable estimate of the quantity and quality of cocaine alkaloid (cocaine base) present in a given sample of cocaine hydrochloride. This is accomplished by removing the HCl molecule (along with most street cuts) and subjecting the resultant cocaine base to a melting point test to determine its purity.

Quantitative

Cocaine hydrochloride is a water-soluble salt whose pH is slightly acidic (6.0). Since the HCl molecule makes up about 11% of the weight, the alkaloid itself can only be 89% of the total. In theory, one gram of pure cocaine hydrochloride, whether illicit or pharmaceutical, will contain 0.89 gram of base. In practice, even with the best lab technique, the conversion to base will result in slight losses caused by some decomposition of the cocaine molecule. A yield of 0.82–0.86 gram indicates a hydrochloride which is practically free of non-baseable adulterants.

In order to estimate the percent of baseable material, the salt is weighed and then dissolved in water. The base is liberated by the slow addition of ammonium hydroxide. This raises the pH of the solution, breaks off the acid molecule, and precipitates cocaine base which is now insoluble in water. The base is separated from the water, dried, and weighed. The dry weight of the base, divided by the weight of the hydrochloride, equals the percent of baseable material.

Qualitative

In addition to the associate coca alkaloids, many substances which are used to adulterate cocaine can convert to bases. Accordingly, an 89% yield does not in itself indicate that the cocaine hydrochloride was pure. If special attention is paid to the way the "cocaine" solution reacts to the cocaine base process, indications of baseable adulterants may be noticed. The melting point is the other important indicator of the purity of the alkaloid.

(Continued on page 112)

WARNING!

Some of the procedures documented, especially those involving volatile solvents or concentrated acids and alkalis may be extremely hazardous. The reader is cautioned not to perform any of thcsc procedures. The procedures described should only be performed under laboratory conditions by professional chemists operating under the authority of the proper government regulatory agencies.

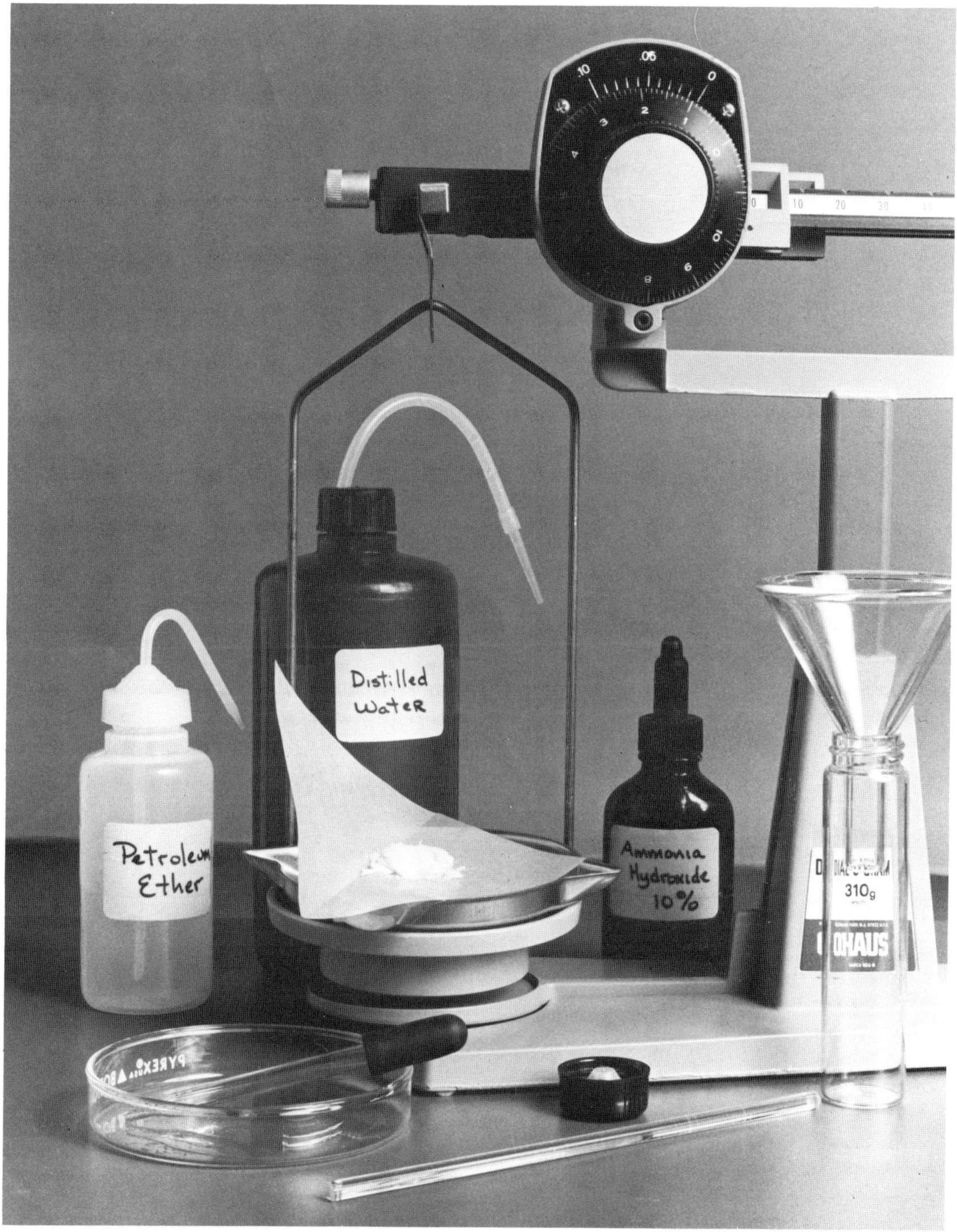

70. Equipment for the cocaine base test includes: petroleum ether (b.p. 35°-60°C) in plastic wash bottle, distilled water in plastic wash bottle, ammonium hydroxide (10% solution in water) in glass dropper bottle, glass powder funnel, 30ml shaker-vial, leakproof cap with polyethylene liner for vial, 6-inch glass stirring rod, 3½-inch glass Petri dish, glass eyedropper, beam balance accurate to 0.01g, glassine weighing paper, sample.

Cocaine is a very weak base which requires a minimum of alkali to precipitate it from its water solution. A single drop of ammonium hydroxide is sufficient to produce a white precipitate; when vigorously stirred the solution becomes milky. Within a few minutes, the solution will begin to clear as the base forms crystals. Further addition of ammonia should produce a similar reaction until the pH of the water is about 7.6. At this point, a drop of ammonia will not produce a visible white precipitate since all the cocaine has been liberated.

Cocaine which contains hygrine, or has been adulterated with a stronger base like lidocaine, will require more alkali for complete precipitation. A single drop of ammonia will produce a visible white precipitate which becomes milky when stirred. However, the base will not separate from the water as crystals, and the solution will therefore remain milky. It requires additional ammonia before separation occurs and the water clarifies. By the time all the base has been liberated, the pH of the water will be 8 or higher.

While the salts of many baseable adulterants have melting points close to that of cocaine, the bases often melt at temperatures which are quite different.

Pharmaceutical cocaine base will melt at 96–98°C. It contains no other alkaloids to lower the temperature.

Uncut illicit cocaine base, which may be as much as 90–95% cocaine, will melt at 92–95°C. There should be no capillary reaction at temperatures below 90°C.

Uncut Potpourri cocaine base, which is rarely over 80% cocaine, will melt at 89–92°C. The presence of cocamine (melting point approximately 80°C.) or hygrine causes a capillary reaction below 90°C.

When lidocaine is present in any of the above bases, the first reaction can occur as low as 60°C. and certainly below 80°C. Most likely the entire melt will be complete before the temperature reaches 90°C.

While the results vary depending on the substance which is causing the deviation, it is obvious when the base is not pure. An experienced tester can make a fairly accurate estimation of the percent of cocaine alkaloid which is present.

As with the melting point test, practice makes perfect. Novices at testing are usually so unsure of their technique that if a test fails they think that it was due to their error. Only experience will make this uncertainty disappear. Perhaps it was not the technique but the *lack* of cocaine which made the test fail.

An accurate cocaine base test may be performed with as little as 0.20 gram of cocaine hydrochloride. The inexperienced tester, however, may find that 0.50–1.00 grams is an easier amount with which to maintain accuracy. A reliable test depends on exacting technique and the use of a scale which is accurate to within 1/100 of a gram.

(Continued on page 123)

COCAINE BASE TEST: Problems and Remedies

INDICATION	CAUSE	REMEDY
The sample of cocaine is not totally soluble in water.	The sample contains a water-insoluble substance; e.g., local anesthetic in base form.	The solution is filtered to remove the insoluble part.
Adding ammonia does not produce a visible white precipitate.	The sample does not contain cocaine hydrochloride.	There is no remedy, but a methyl benzoate test should be done to confirm or deny the presence of cocaine.
A visible white reaction occurs but no precipitate is formed.	There are two possibilities: 1. The cocaine is overly acidic, requiring more ammonia to precipitate the base. 2. The base which is precipitating is not cocaine but an oil like hygrine or procaine.	1. More ammonia is added; close attention is paid to the pH so excess ammonia is not added. 2. The crystals are extracted at the point that ammonia precipitates only oily material.
A precipitate is formed which is insoluble in petroleum ether.	The precipitate is not cocaine base.	The precipitate is separated by filtration and examined and returned to vendor.
The base weight is greater than the hydrochloride.	The base is not dry.	The drying procedure is continued until weight ceases to change.

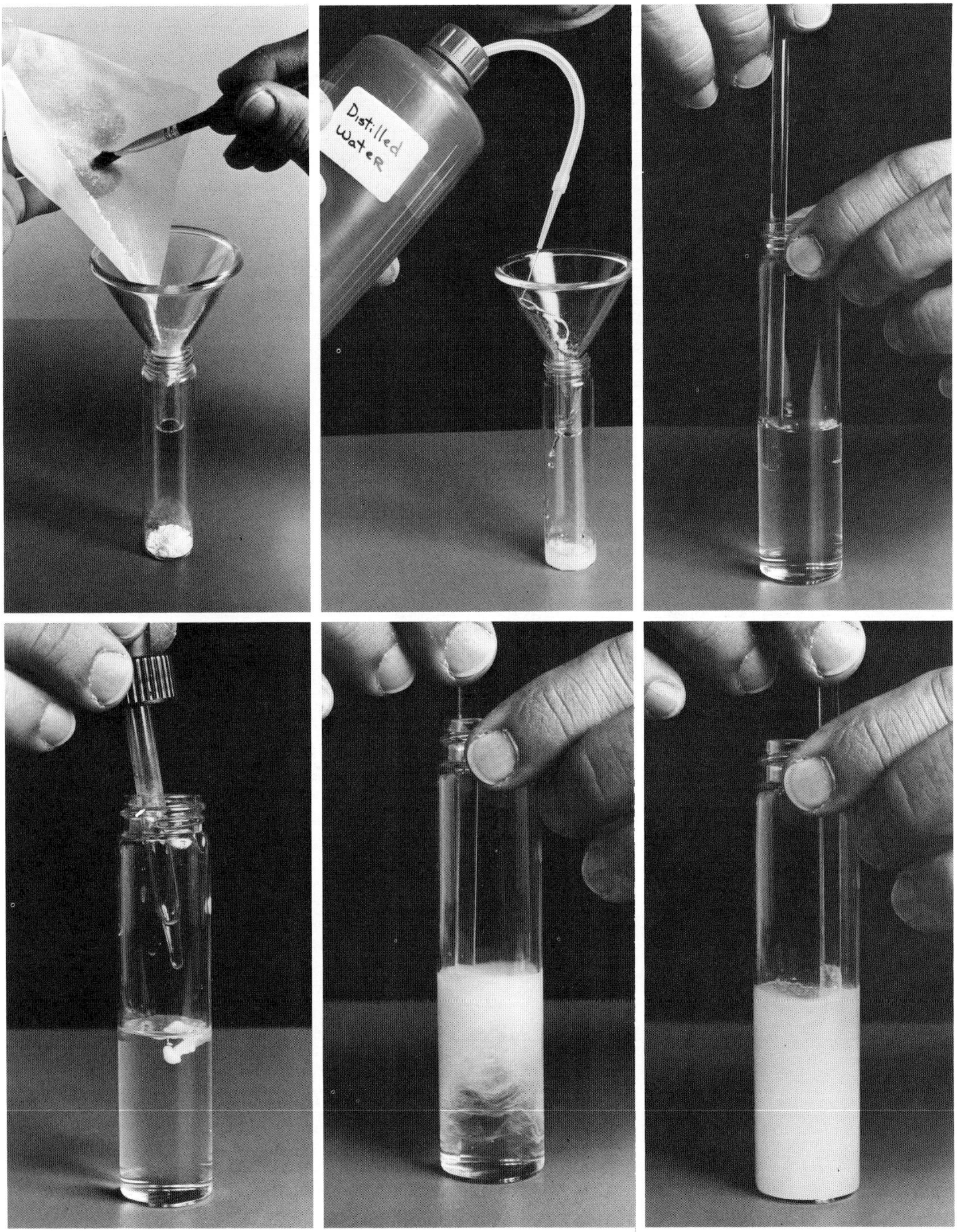

top row, left to right:

71. The sample, weighing 0.5g, is transferred into the vial. The last traces are brushed into the funnel.
72. The water is added, washing all traces into the shaker vial. (For 0.5g of sample, 10-15ml of water is used.)
73. The water is stirred to completely dissolve the sample.

bottom row, left to right:

74. A single drop of ammonium hydroxide solution produces a white precipitate.
75. Stirring produces a milky solution.
76. After one minute, crystals start forming and the solution begins to clear.

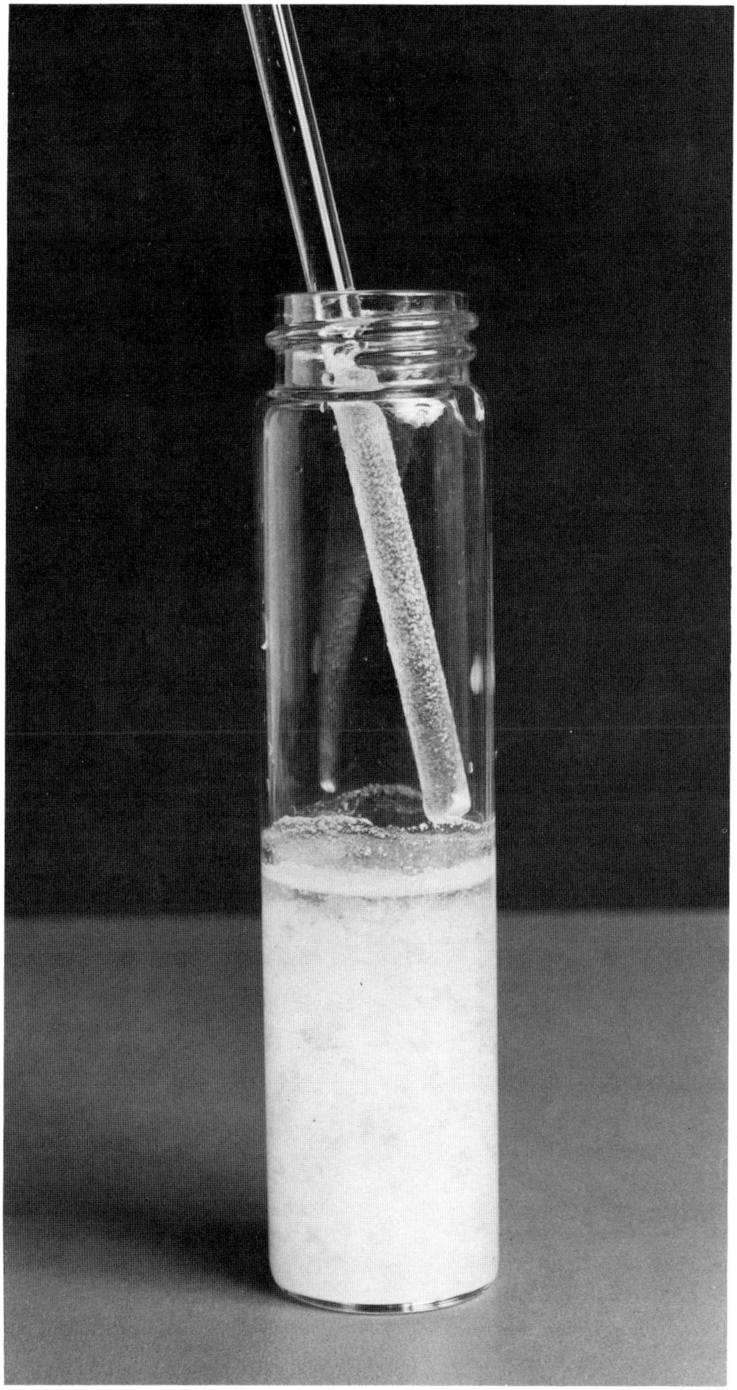

77. If the sample is pure cocaine, crystals of cocaine base are deposited on the rod and side of the vial. The solution clears as the crystals fall to the bottom.

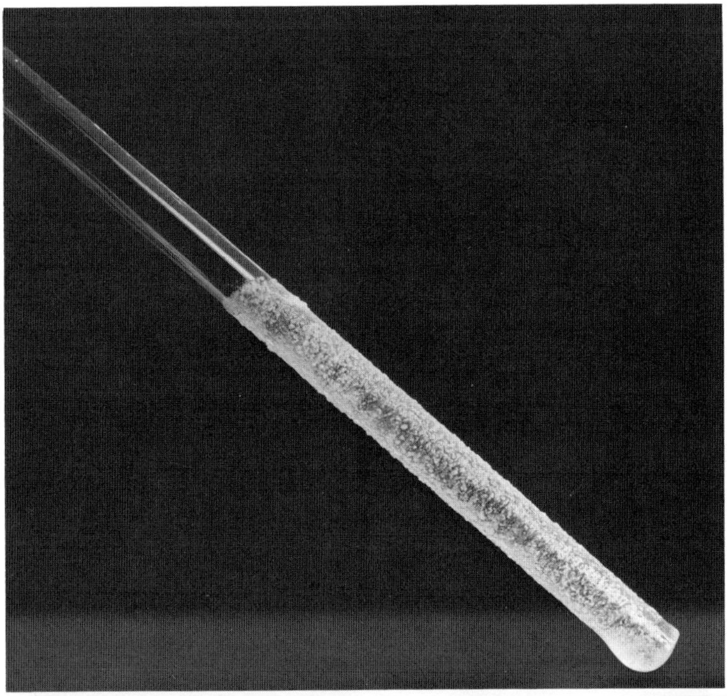

78. A close-up of the stirring rod.

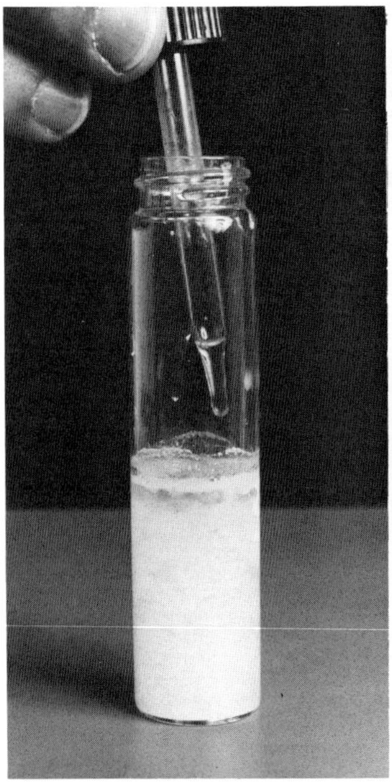

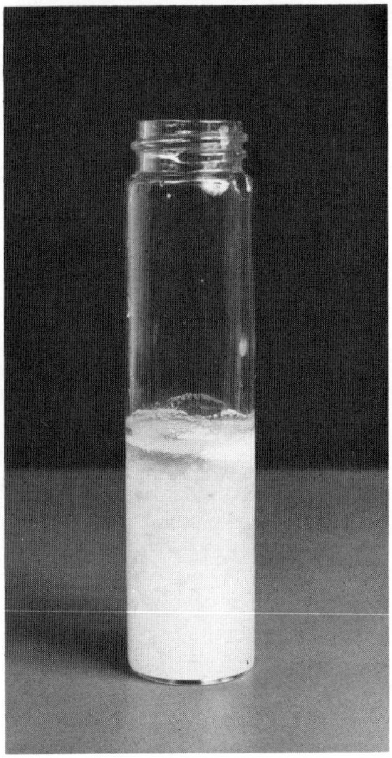

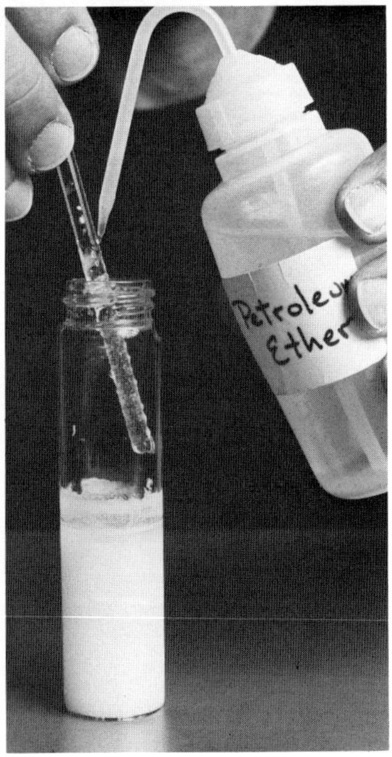

79. Additional drops of ammonium hydroxide solution are added until the pH reaches 7.6.
80. Here additional precipitation is seen.
81. After precipitation is complete, traces of cocaine base are washed into the vial with petroleum ether.

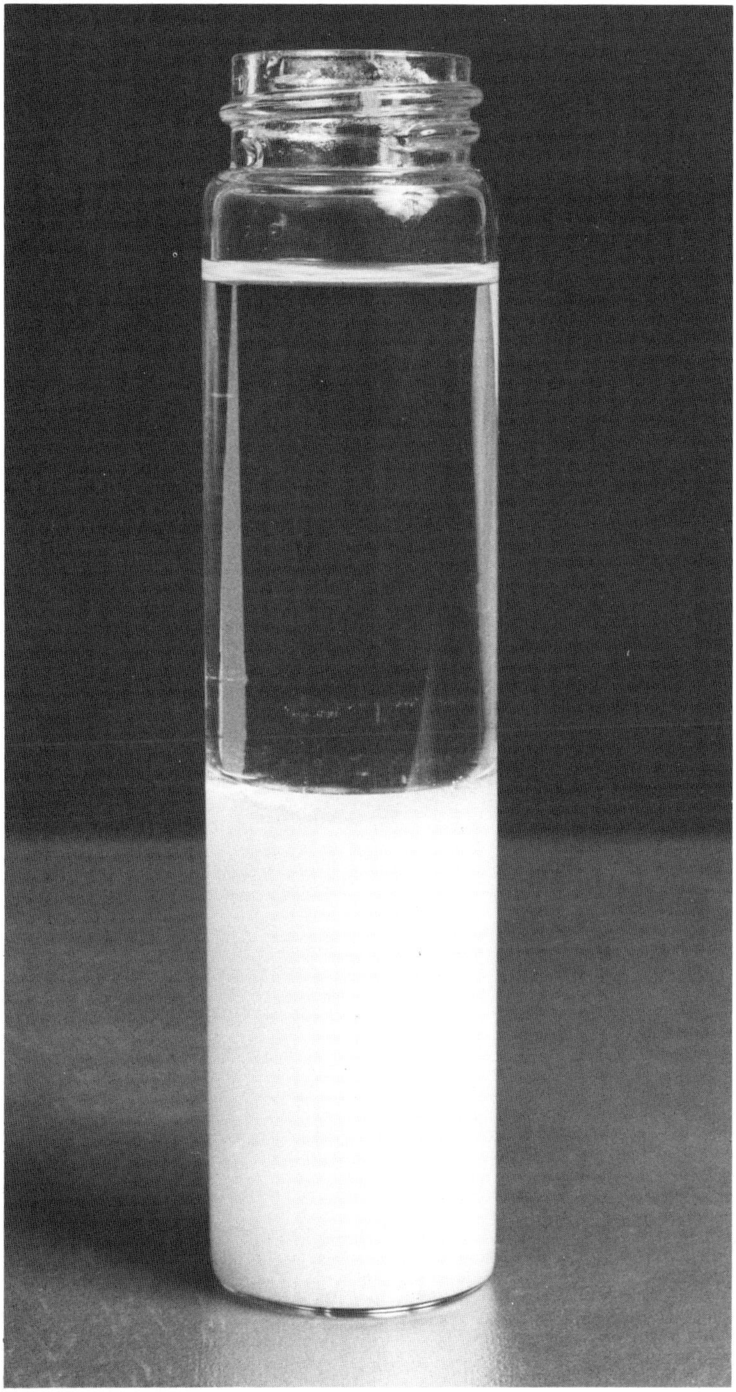

82. More petroleum ether is added until the amount equals that of the water.

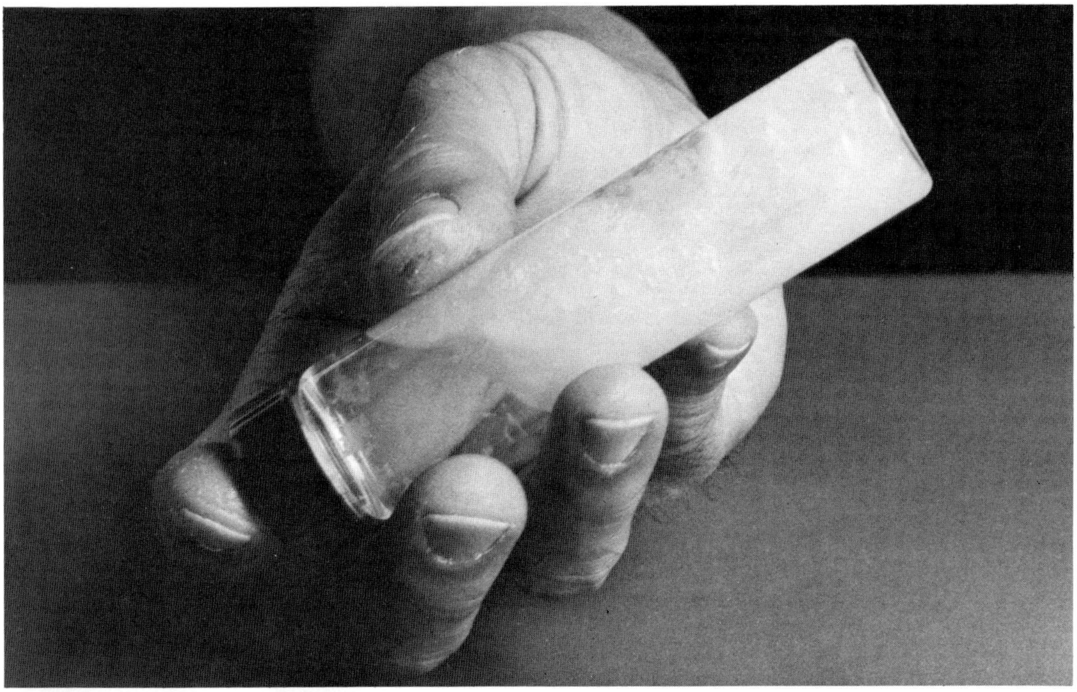

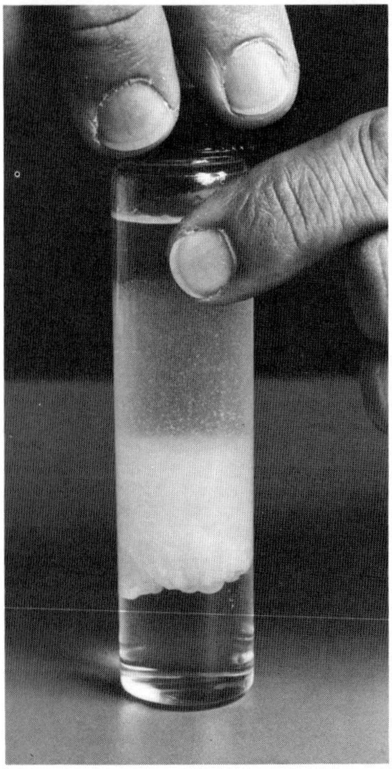

83. The vial is inverted and shaken vigorously for 30 seconds. The petroleum ether dissolves the cocaine base crystals.

84. The cap is opened slightly to release the pressure. The water and petroleum ether separate into layers.

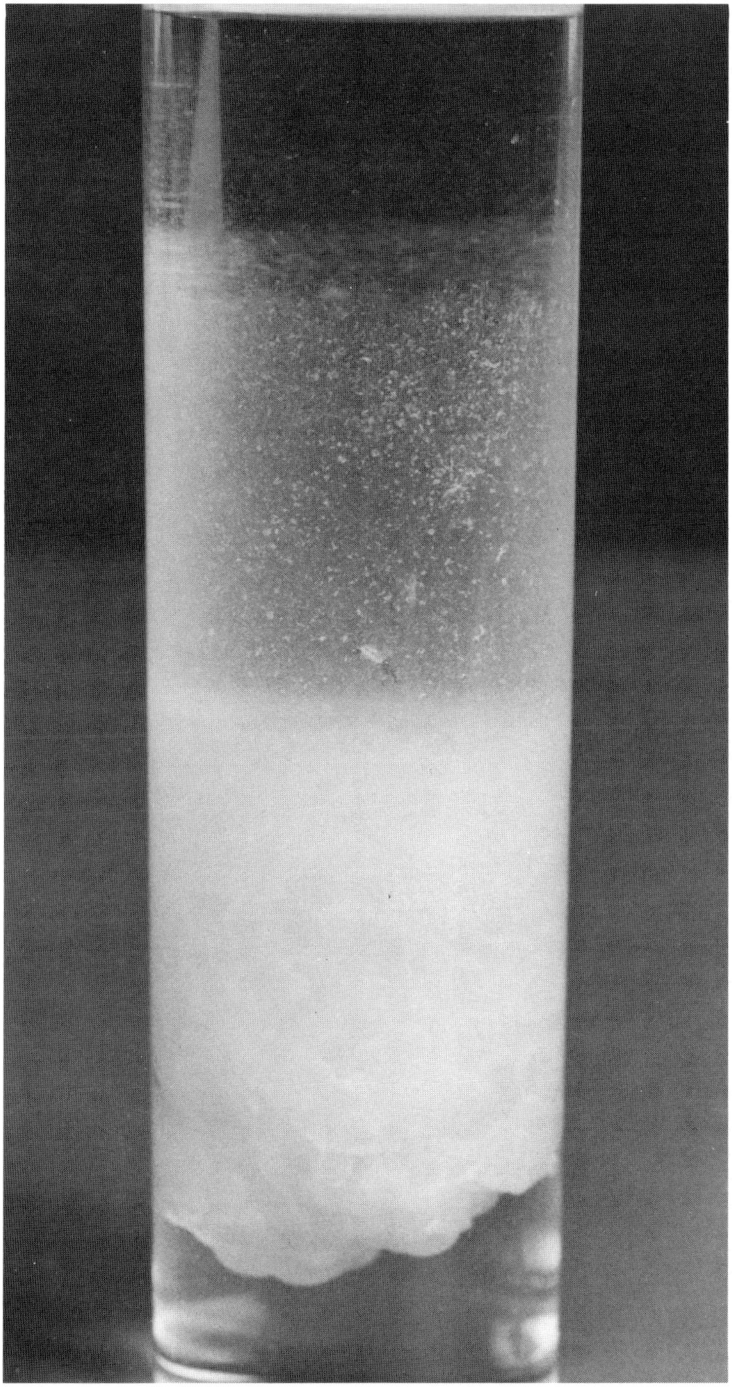

85. After that first extraction, some crystals remain, indicating that the petroleum ether is saturated and can dissolve no more cocaine base.

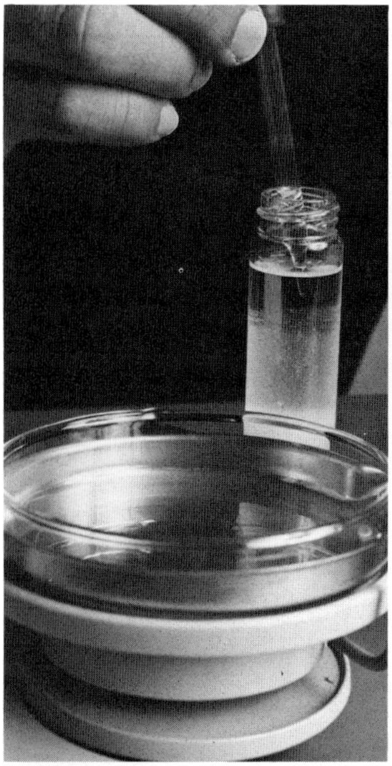
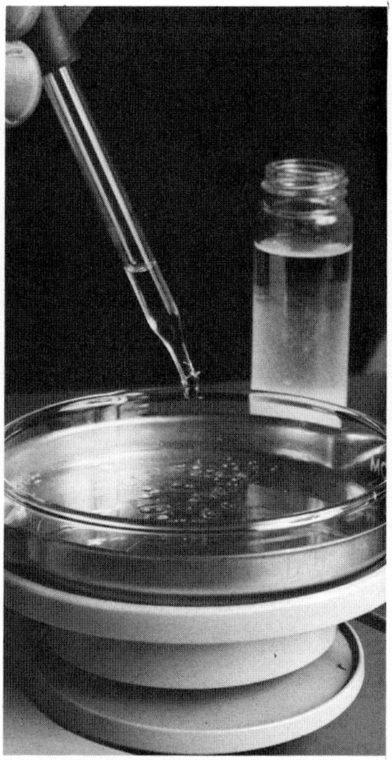
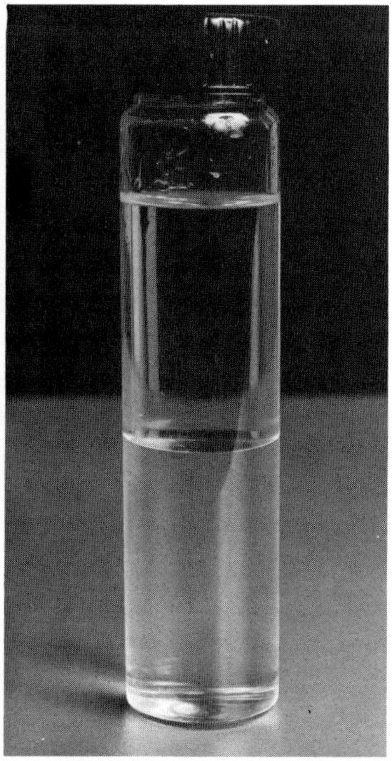
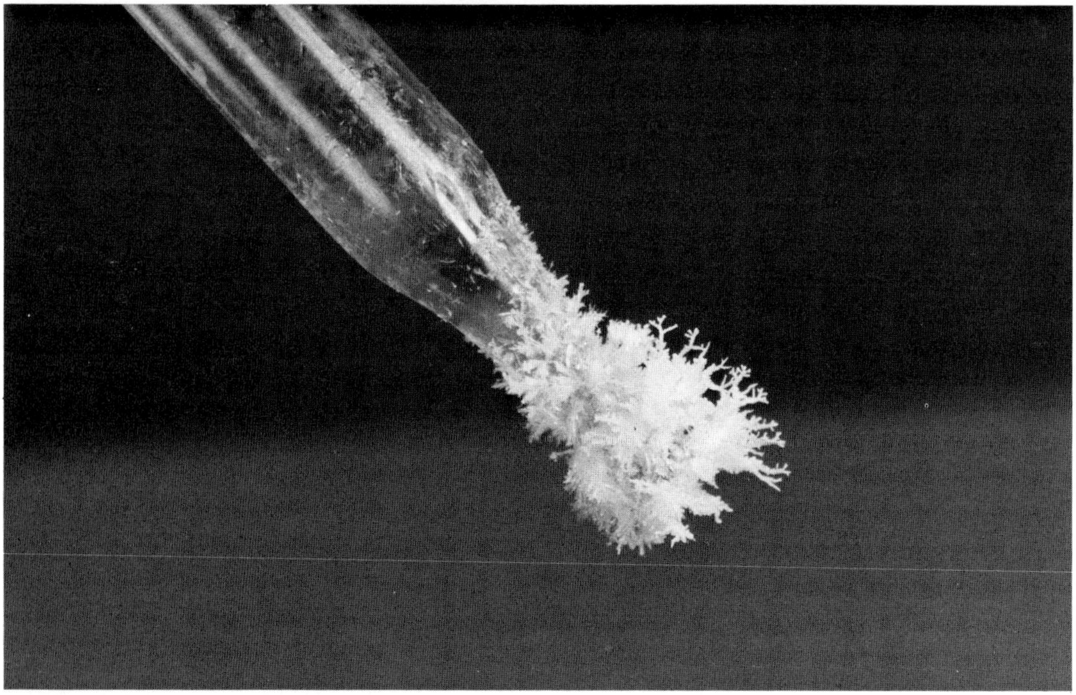

top row:

86. The petroleum ether layer (top) is removed with an eyedropper. Care is taken not to remove any of the water layer.
87. The petroleum ether is transferred to the pre-weighed Petri dish on a scale.
88. After the third extraction, all the cocaine base crystals have dissolved.

bottom:

89. Crystals grow on the tip of the eyedropper due to the rapid evaporation of the petroleum ether.

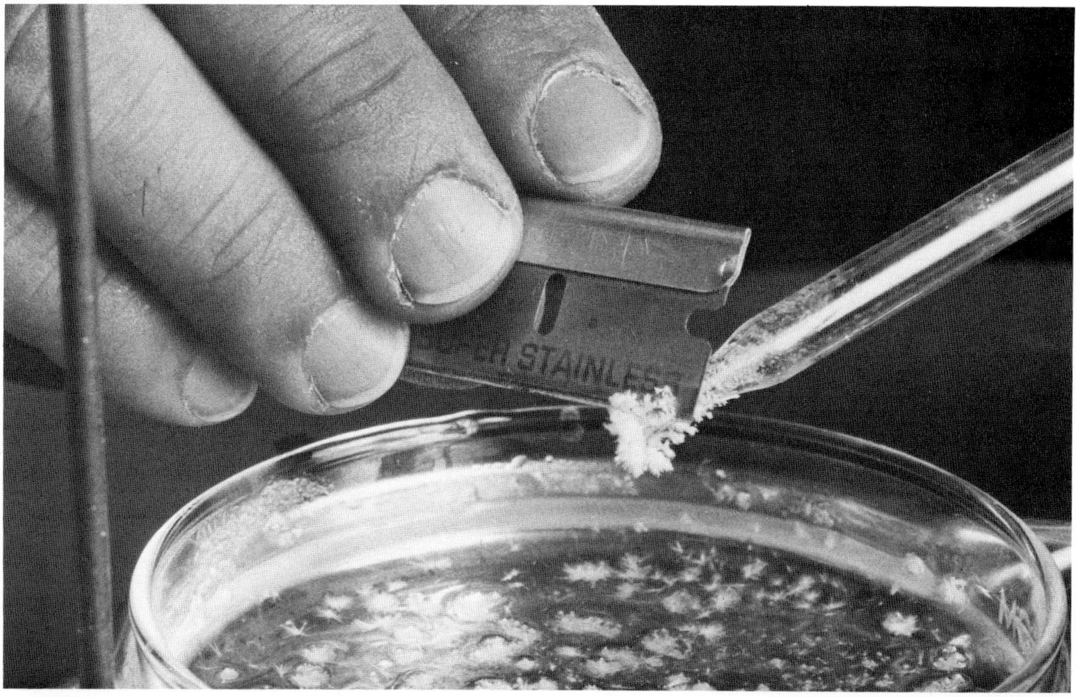

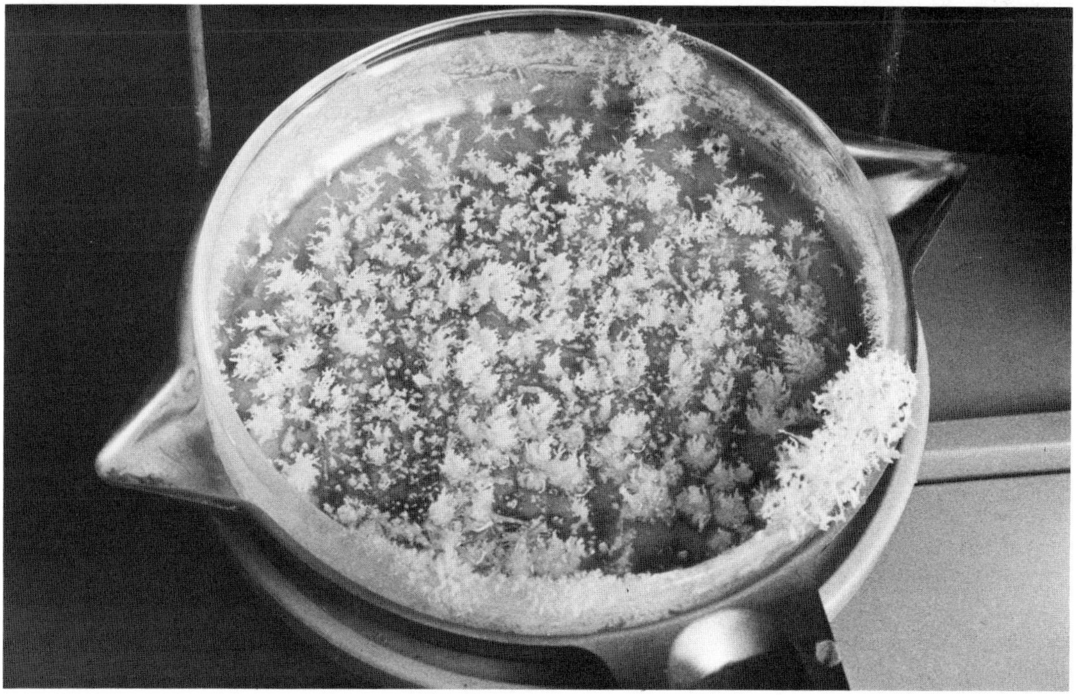

90. Care is taken to recover all the weight; even eyedropper is scraped. (It can also be rinsed off with petroleum ether.)

91. After the petroleum ether has totally evaporated, 0.43g of cocaine base crystals remain in the Petri dish. This is 86% of the original 0.50g, indicating that the sample was relatively free of non-baseable cuts.

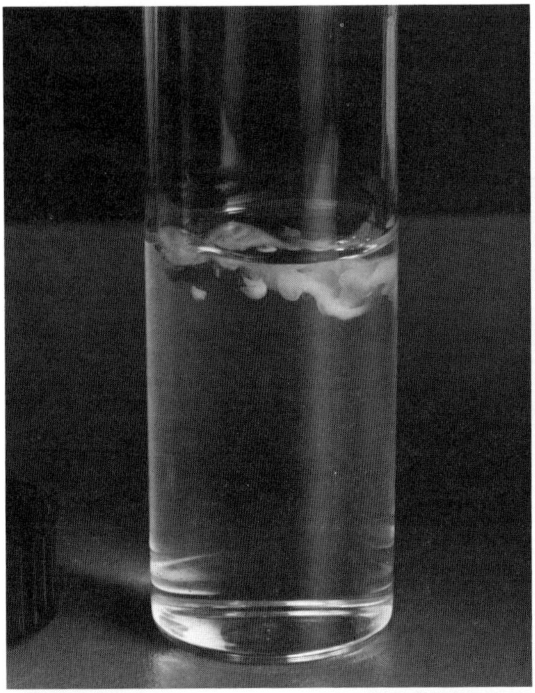

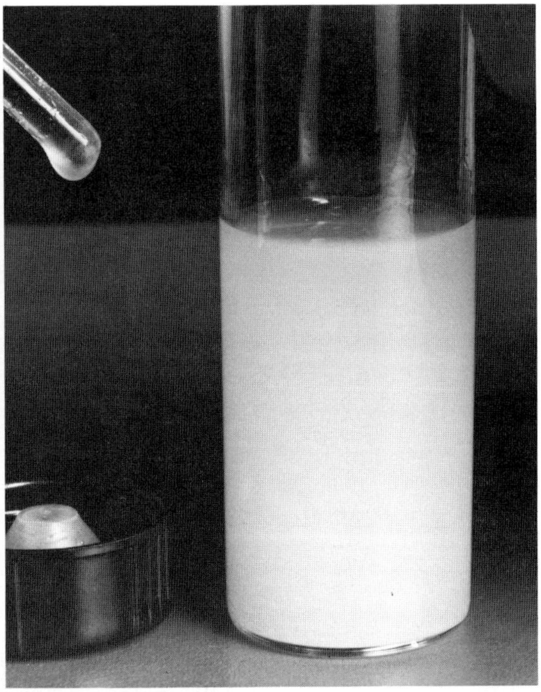

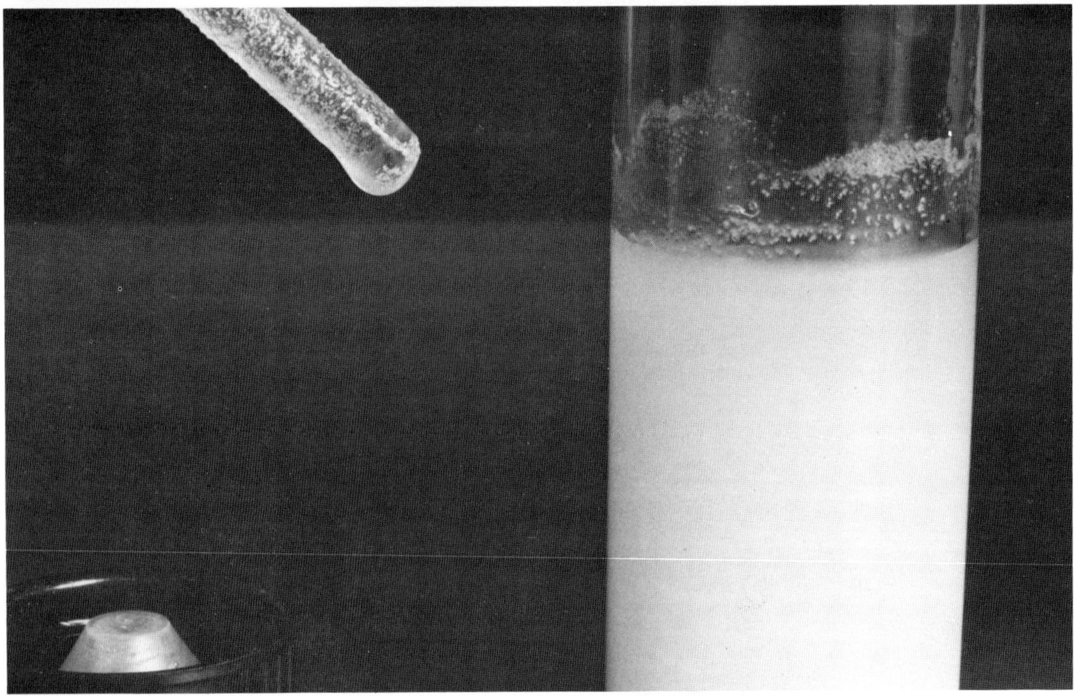

top:

92. When the same sample is cut with 25% lidocaine, the first drop produces the same reaction as in photo 74, p. 114.
93. But after several minutes of stirring, no crystals appear on stirring rod or side of vial; the solution remains milky. (Compare to the clearing solution of photo 77, p. 115.)

bottom:

94. After two drops of the ammonium hydroxide solution, crystals form on rod and side of vial, but the solution remains milky. With pure cocaine the solution would be clear.

In the Lab

To the professional chemist with access to the most recent technology, the problem of testing for purity and adulterants is almost a trivial one. Whereas the street tests available to the consumer require judgments which might be influenced by some financial loss or gain, the professional systems are based mainly on instrument readings. One might understand the street tester making an error in judgment due to this personal involvement; the professional chemist has no such excuse.

The professionals engaged in lab testing of cocaine are mainly governmental and law enforcement agencies, researchers in universities, drug companies, and some labs licensed by the government to do analysis for the public. Until a few years ago, public analysis labs could legally divulge quantitative as well as qualitative information. An individual submitting a sample could therefore learn not only which compounds were present, but also the exact percentage of each. The logic of discontinuing the percent

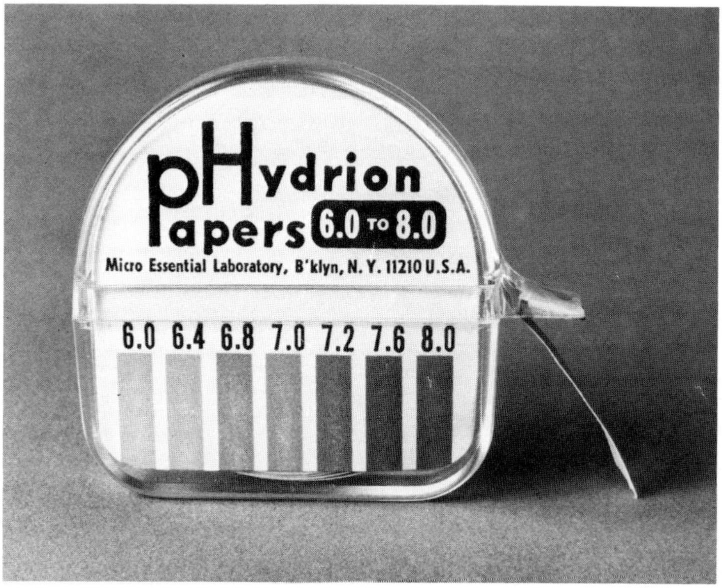

95. Paper used to measure the pH of solutions. The paper is wet with the solution and the resulting color is matched to the color key on the container.

composition report was that it would help drug dealers to test quality and thereby encourage dealing. More likely, however, when the street-level consumer realized that he was being sold 10% cocaine and 90% adulterants at $100 per gram, he would be less likely to throw away his money, not buy the gram, and thereby discourage dealing. On the other hand, being able to sell cheap adulterants to the uninformed public at $100 per gram and realize 500–1000% profit on the cocaine is more likely to encourage new dealers to compromise their integrity in search of a fast buck. Since the budget of the DEA (Drug Enforcement Administration) is proportional to the problems it faces, many jobs are dependent on continued drug traffic. If ever the DEA were able to stop drug dealing, it would remove the reason for its existence. Under the present system, the ironic result is that increased drug traffic benefits both the dealers and the DEA, with the consumer getting the short end from both sides.

The methods used in professional labs vary with the kind of information being sought. While the classical melting points, color reactions, and crystal derivation tests are used, most are only valid if the sample is free of interfering substances, that is, unadulterated. The usual procedure, therefore, is first to separate the sample into its different components and then test for the compounds of interest.

The most sophisticated tools used are a gas chromatograph coupled to a high-resolution mass spectrometer. These provide information about the specific atomic makeup of an unknown molecule. The necessary equipment can cost $50,000 and up. The least expensive, but still sophisticated method, thin-layer chromatography, separates compounds in a mixture from each other. This shows the relative purity of the sample. When coupled to a spectrophotometer, a percentage can be estimated. Thin-layer chromatography equipment can cost less than $100, but the spectrophotometer is in the $1000 range.

Forensic labs need information which can be provided with the less expensive equipment since they are only concerned with a few *illegal* substances. The researchers interested in the chemistry of the mother plant or in the chemistry of the drug after it has been ingested by an animal may need the information about all the other (and possibly previously undiscovered) compounds present. For this kind of information, the most sophisticated system may be necessary.

Laboratory studies done on the effects of cocaine on animals and humans are *necessarily* done with pure cocaine. The regulations on human experimentation are very strict, so using street cocaine in any such study would be virtually impossible. The reality, then, is that the few experiments done under controlled conditions may miss much of the physiological and psychological effects of the cocaine most people use—in particular, the possible interaction of other alkaloids which may produce different types of highs. Whether these variations are the result of different dosages, the presence of other alkaloids, or added adulterants, is at this point unclear; everyone with first-hand experience has his own opinion of what is happening. Considering the 10 to 20 million Americans performing these experiments at an expense of $25 to $50 billion per year, it would seem to merit further attention from medical researchers.

COLOR PLATES

- Coca Plant and Leaves
- Cocaine in Various Forms
- Results of Melting Point and Foil Burn Tests

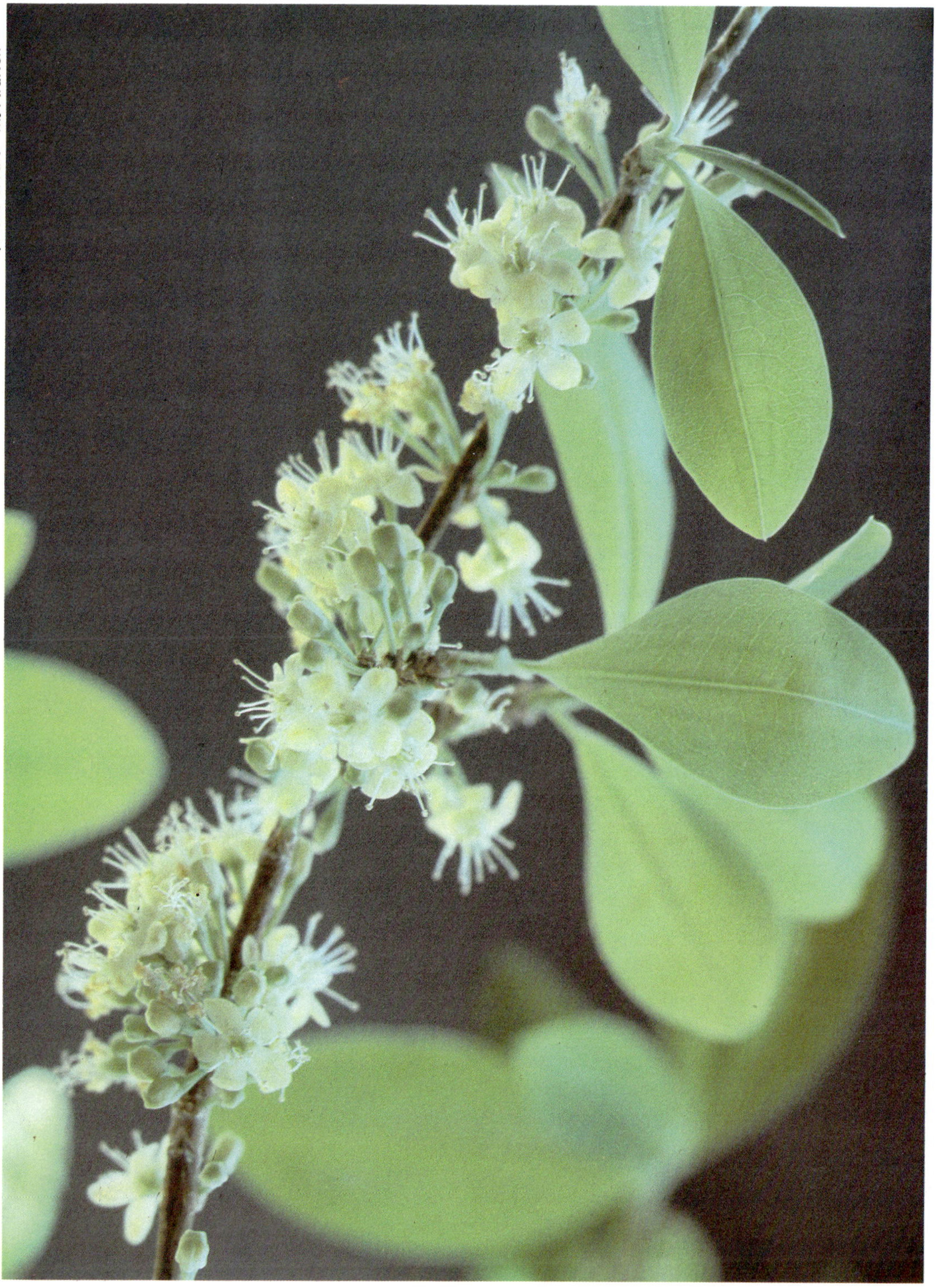

photo credit: M. Aldrich

1. Graceful blossoms on an Erythroxylum coca plant. The two lines parallel to the midrib, characteristic of coca, are visible on the large leaf at the center.

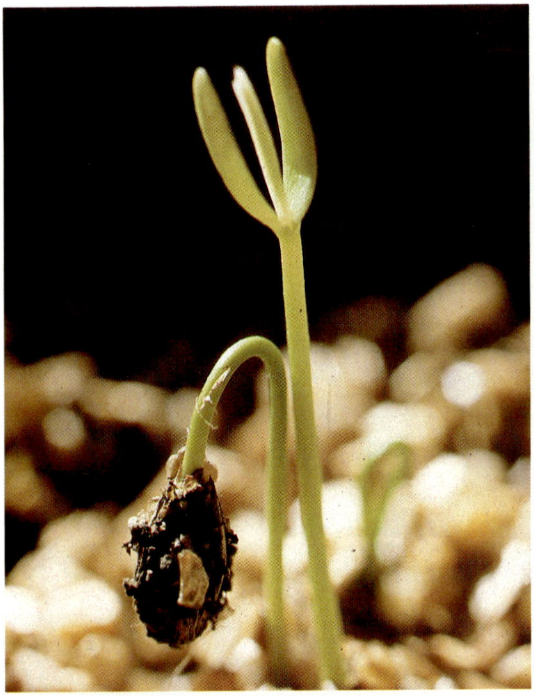

photo credit: M. Aldrich

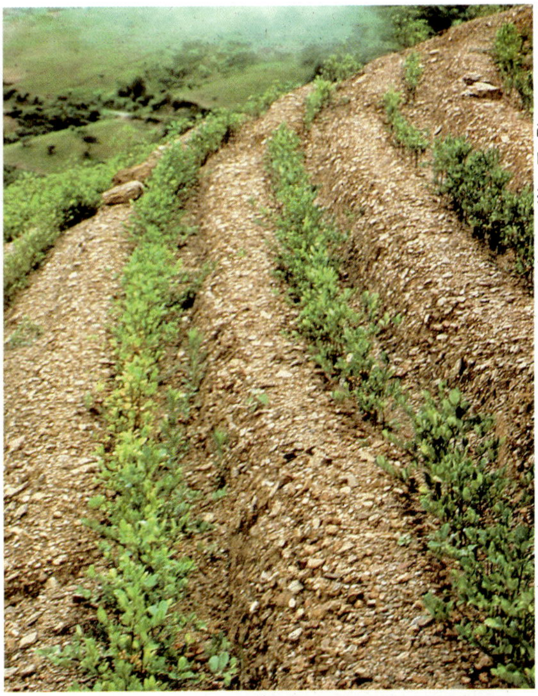

photo credit: T. Plowman

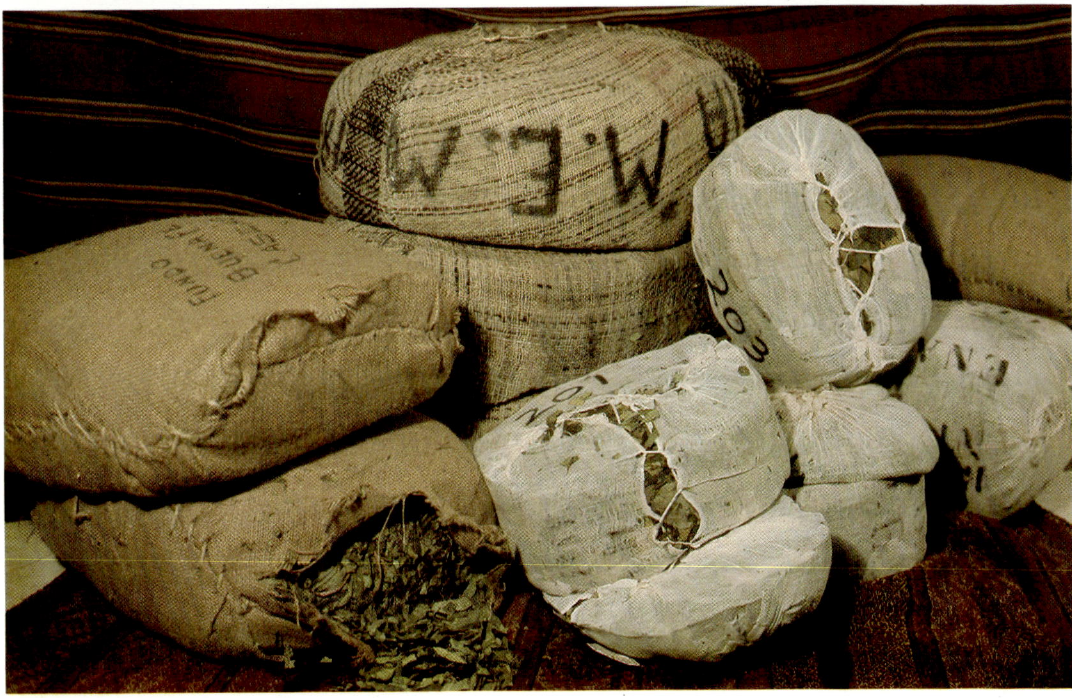

photo credit: C.W. Greene

2. (top left) **Fragile two-week-old coca sprouts, showing development of dicotyledons.**

3. (top right) **Plantation of E. coca in the Bolivian Yungas.**

4. (bottom) **Bales of coca leaves shipped from various locations in the Andes to the Harvard Botanical Museum (for research purposes).**

5. (at right) **A bale from Cuzco, Peru (probably E. coca) has been opened and the leaves are being inspected.**
6. (below) **Various leaves and alkalis with chuspa (coca pouch).**

photo credit: C.W. Greene

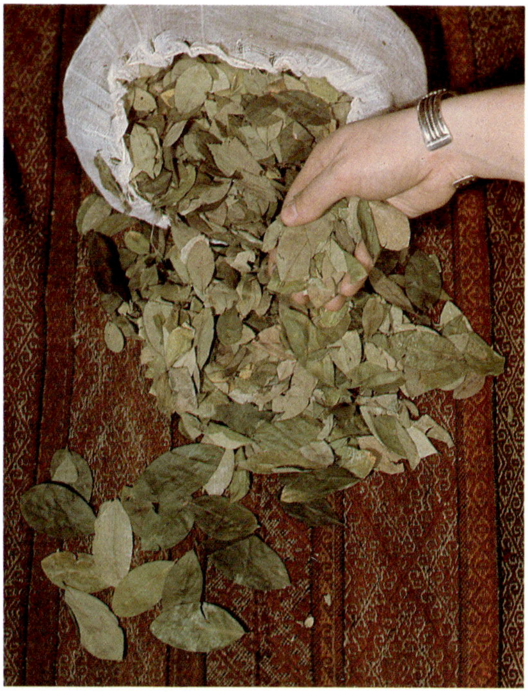

photo credit: C.W. Greene

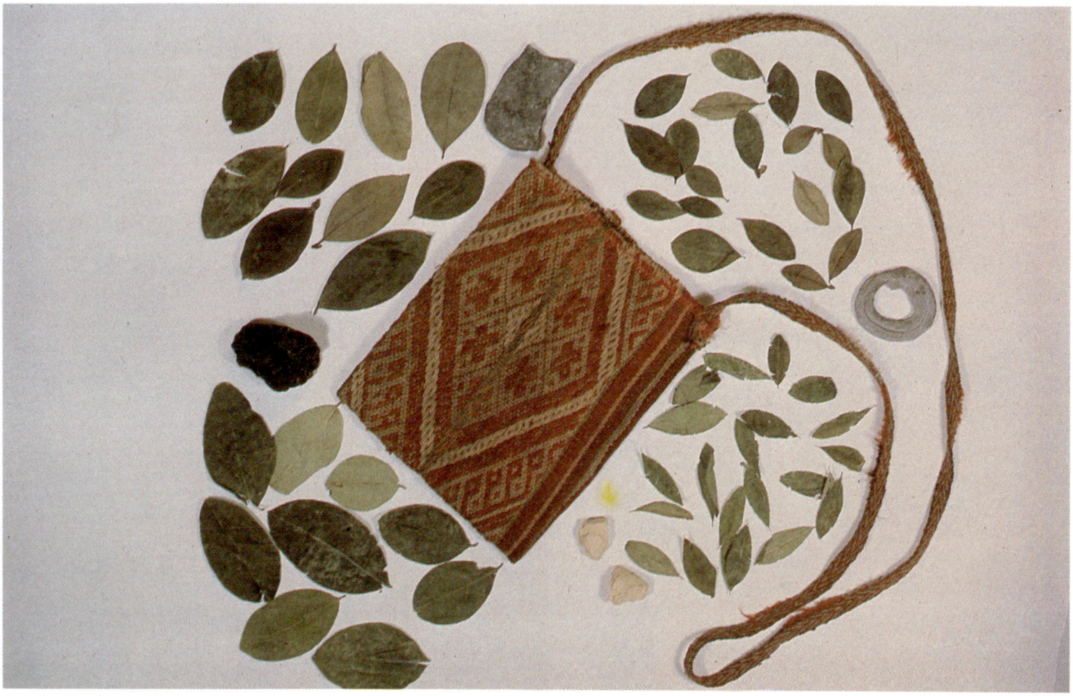

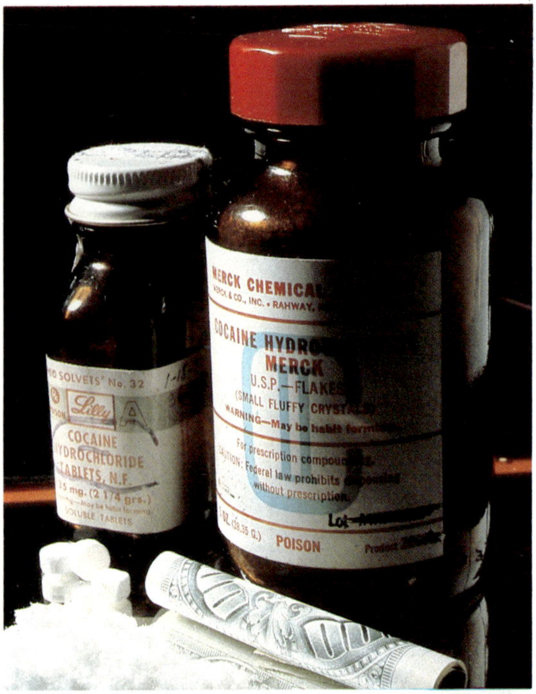

photo credit: J. Bigwood

7. (at left) Two kinds of pharmaceutical cocaine—fluffy crystals of Merck and 135-milligram tablets of Lilly—shown with the bottles in which they are distributed.

8. (below) Peruvian style flake made in Colombia by a master "cook." Cocaine of this quality and appearance is rare in the illicit market.

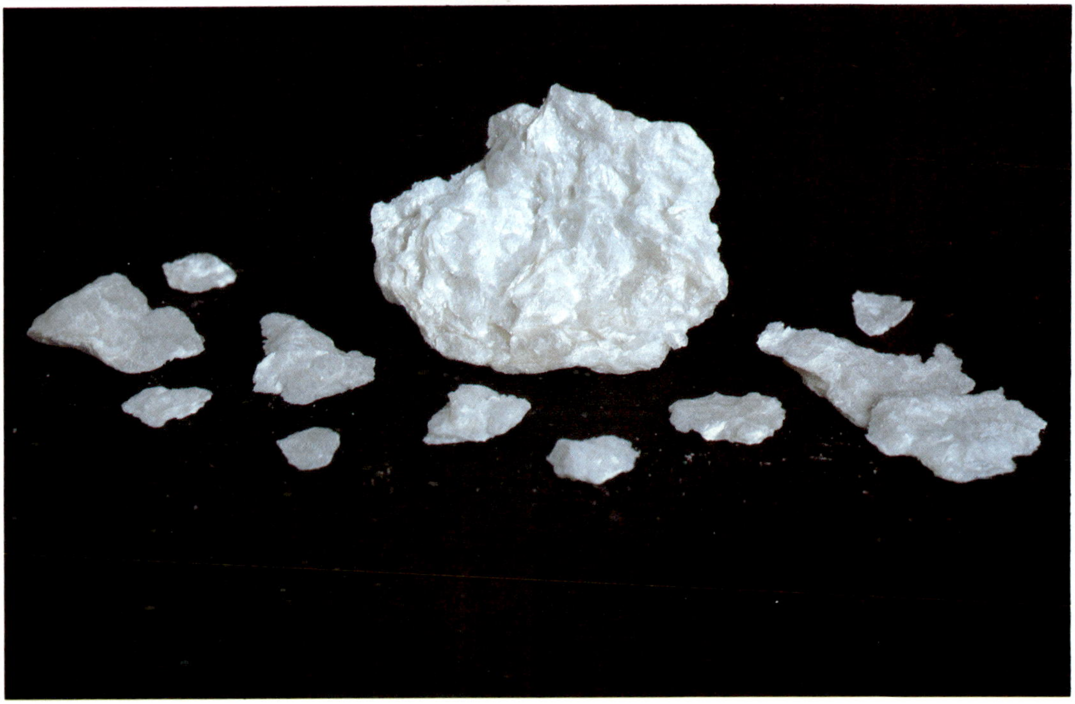

9. (top right) "Bolivian rock" made close to the growing area. The crude refining process, omitting several steps, involved soaking the leaves in lime water, extracting the alkaloids with gasoline, and precipitating the cocaine by adding hydrochloric acid to the gasoline.

10. (middle) Cocaine base made by filtration from the "Bolivian rock" shown in previous photo.

11. (below) The base from color plate 10 produced this 19-gram piece of cocaine hydrochloride after it was crystallized out of diethyl ether.

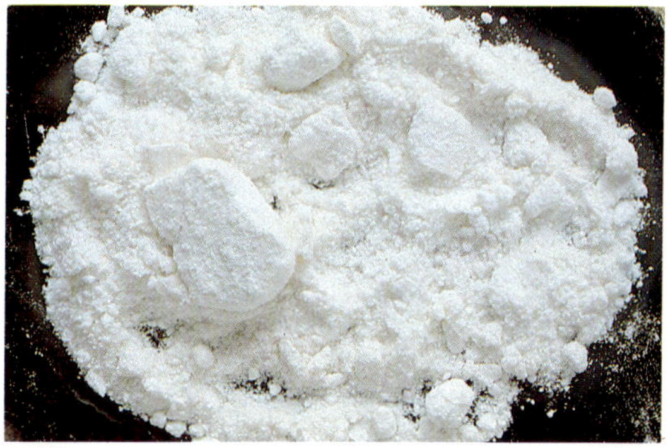

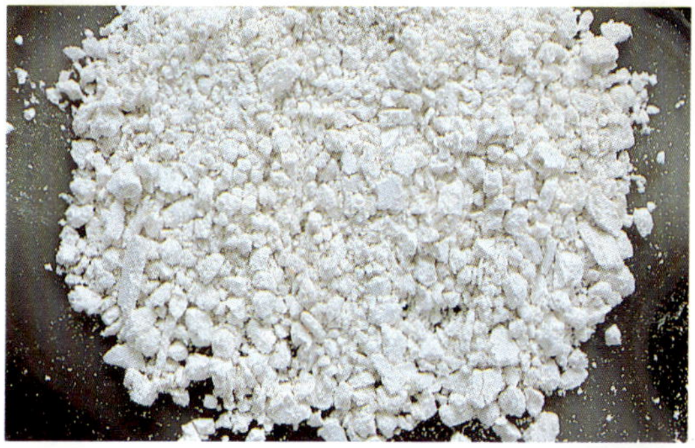

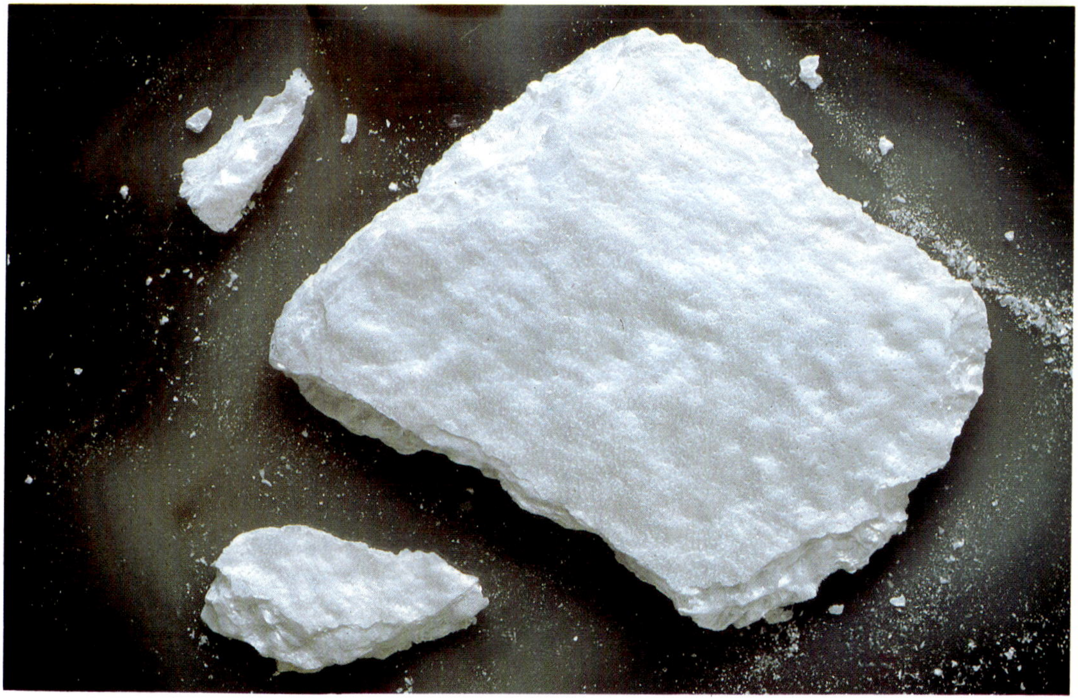

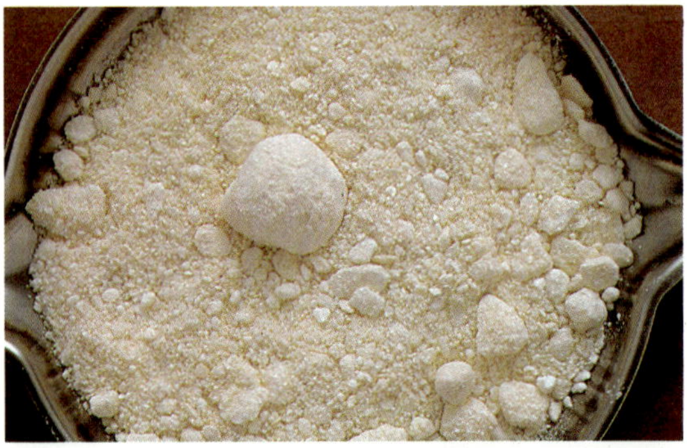

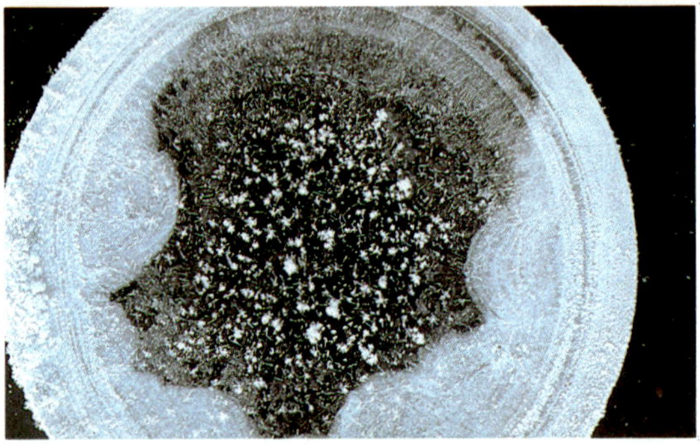

12. (top left) "Potpourri" cocaine made in Colombia by combining pasta of varied quality from many growing regions. This commonly seen form usually contains less than 50% cocaine and includes hygrine, cocamine, benzoylecgonine and other impurities.

13. (middle) Crystals of cocaine base made from the "potpourri" shown above by extraction with petroleum ether.

14. This broken disc of vacuum-filtered cocaine hydrochloride flakes was made from the base shown above in color plate 13. South American "cooks" say that the vacuum destroys the crystal structure necessary to make flake. Therefore, this was dubbed the "impossible flake."

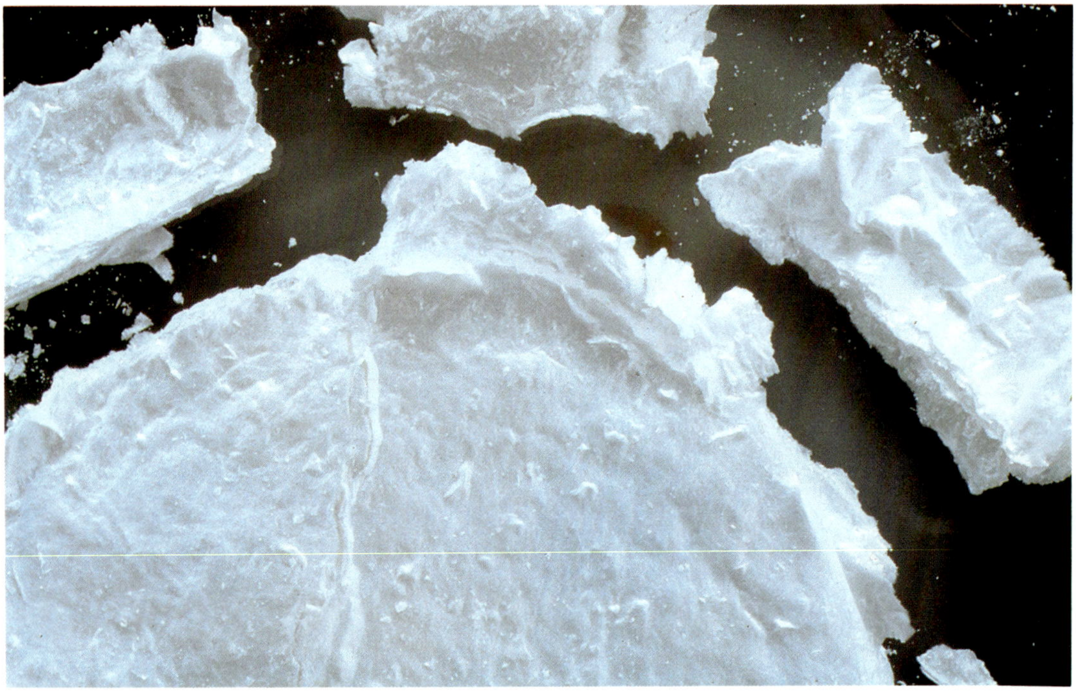

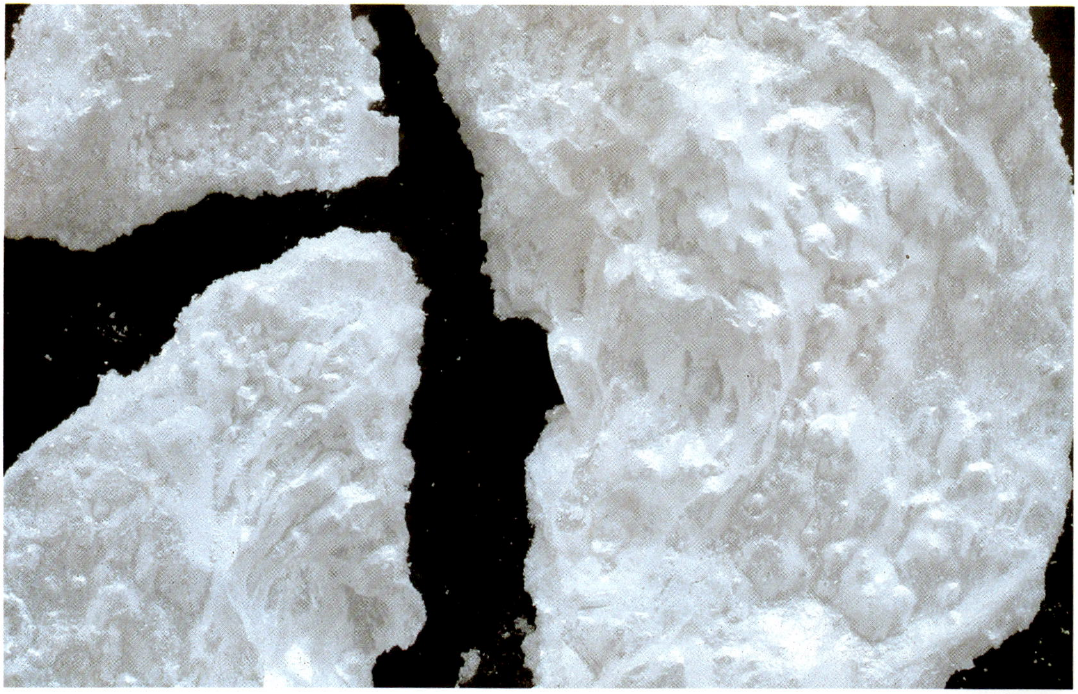

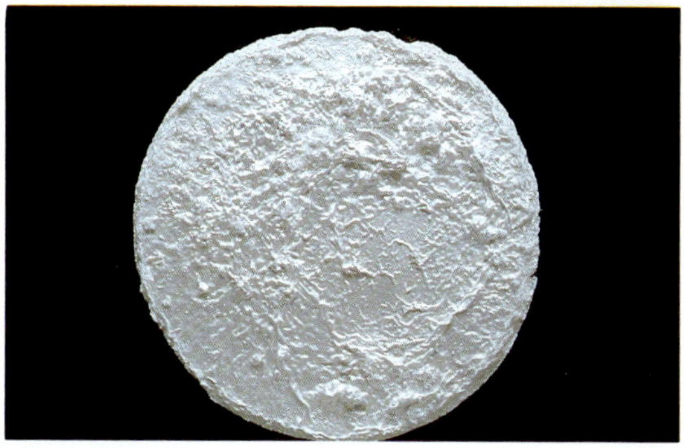

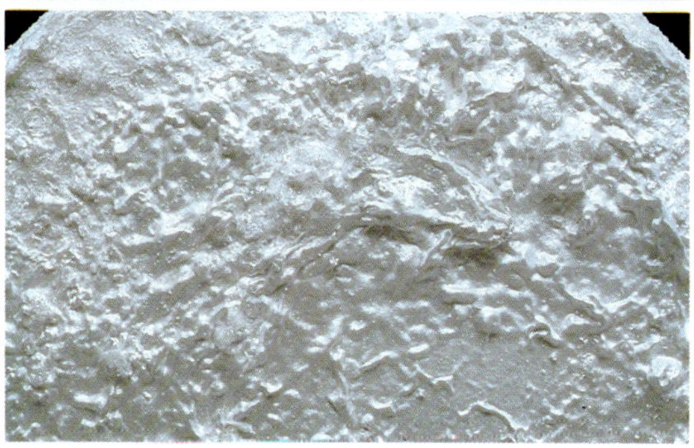

15. (above) **Cocaine hydrochloride "made in USA" using base imported from South America. The use of quality chemicals and proper technique yields a more refined product.**

16. (right) **Fifty-gram "moon disc" of cocaine made from the same imported base. The circular shape was formed by the funnel during vacuum filtration.**

17. (lower right) **Detail of the "moon disc" surface, showing the clumps of larger crystals.**

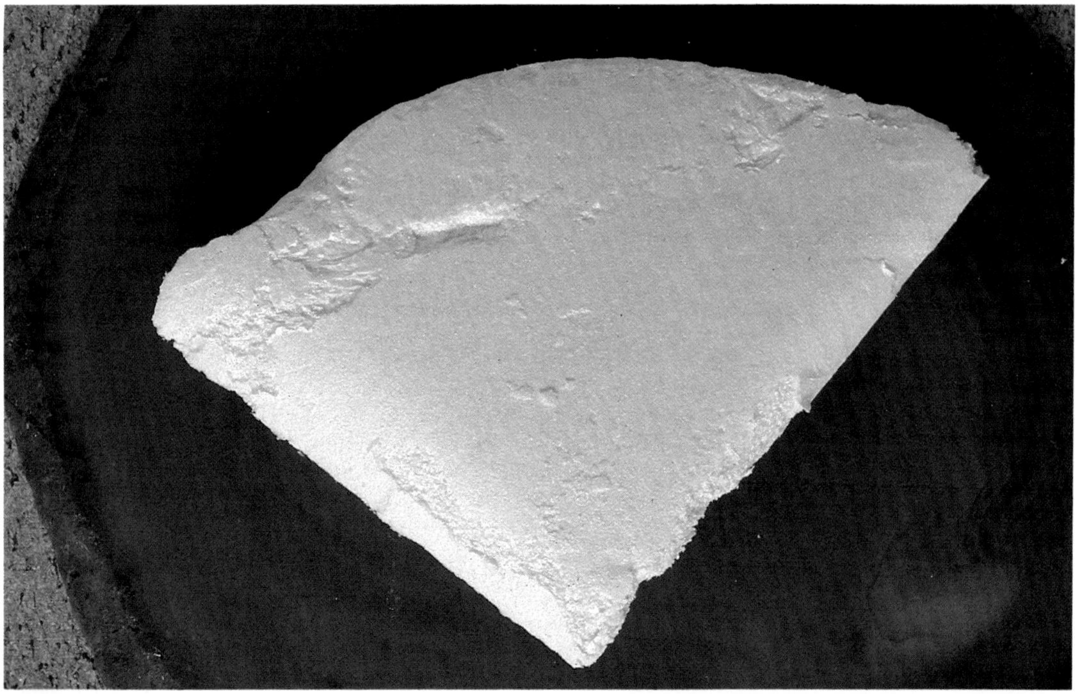

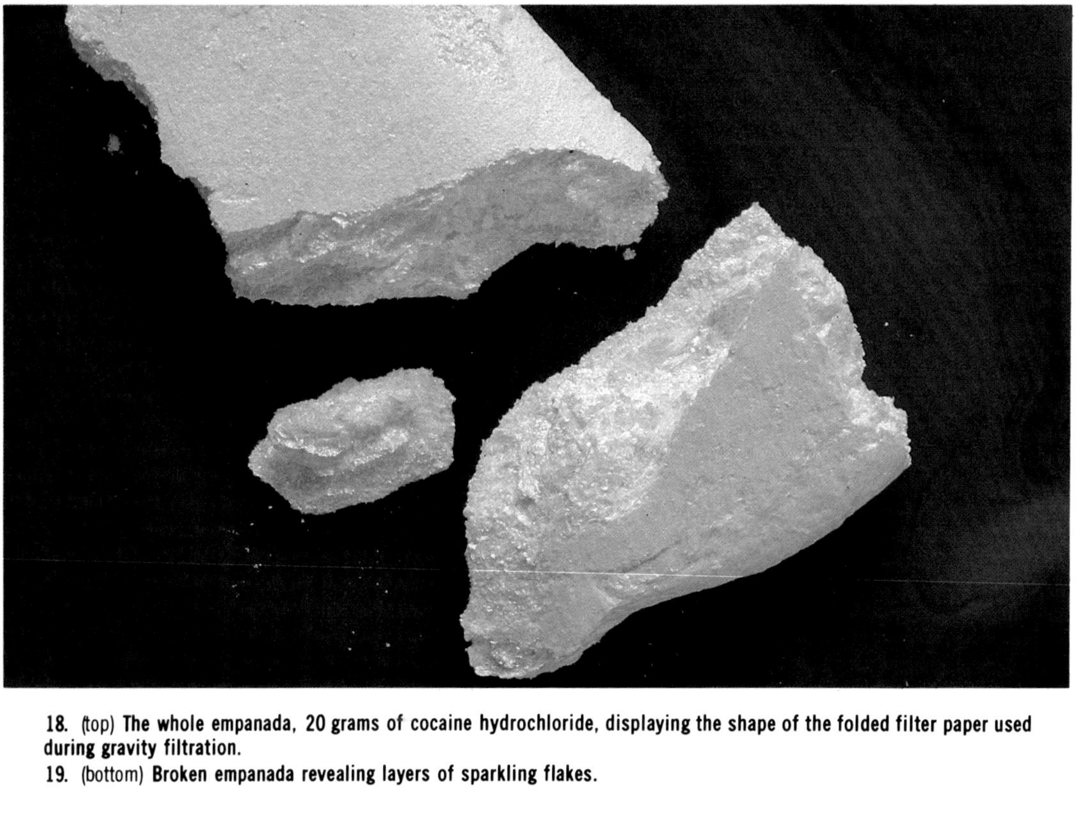

18. (top) The whole empanada, 20 grams of cocaine hydrochloride, displaying the shape of the folded filter paper used during gravity filtration.
19. (bottom) Broken empanada revealing layers of sparkling flakes.

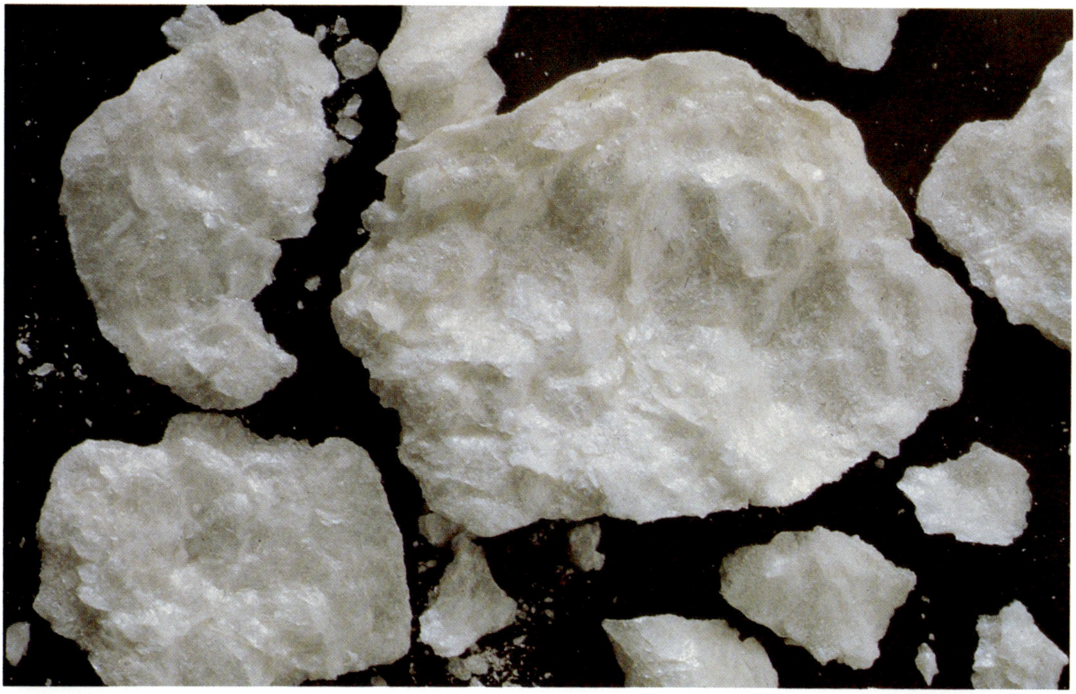

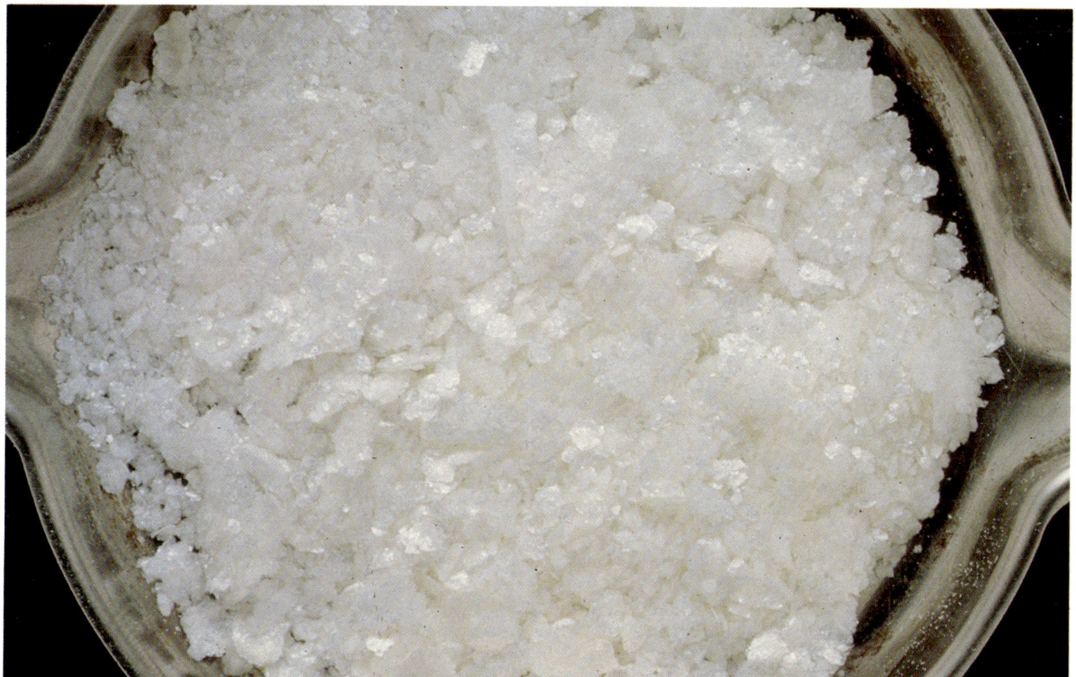

20. (top) This imported flake, also shown in color plate 8, contained hygrine and excess acid.
21. (bottom) After an acetone wash, much of the hygrine and excess acid were removed. This procedure also removed much of the yellow discoloration.

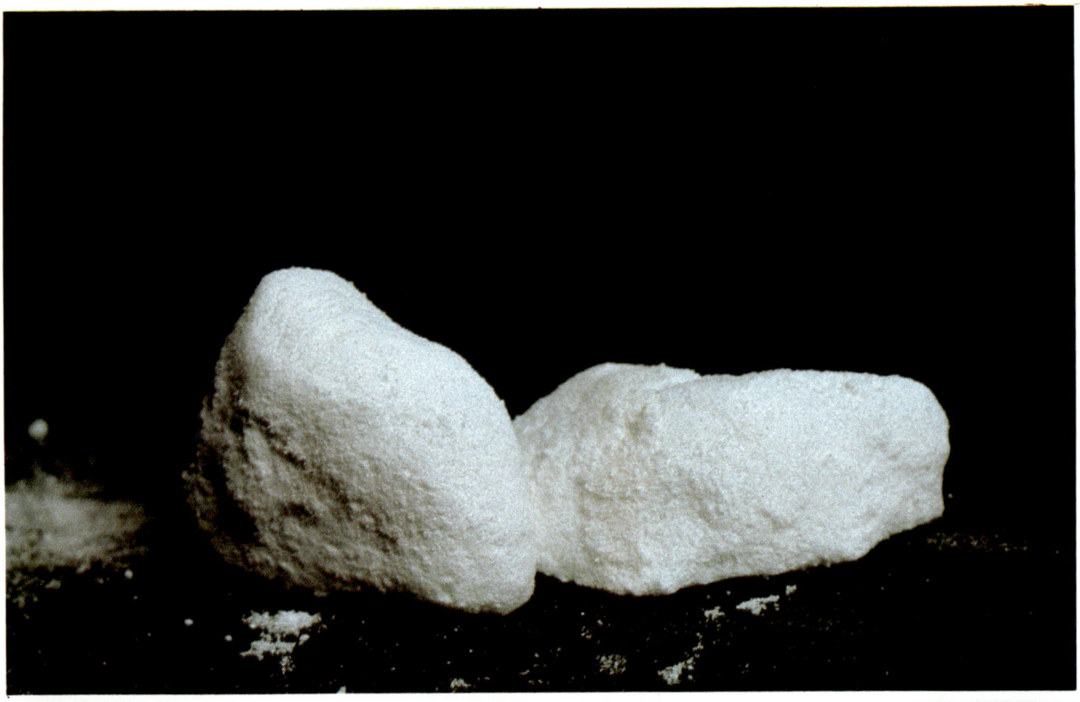

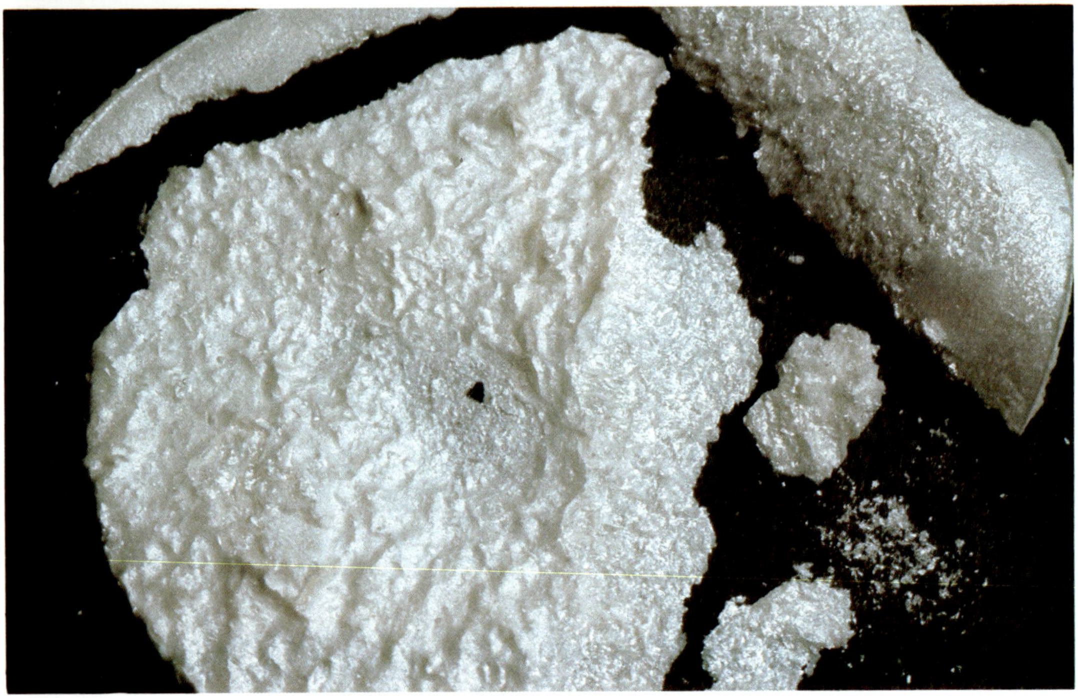

22. (top) Cocaine reconstituted with a non-baseable adulterant, mannitol. This was detected when two melting points were observed during the melting point test (165°C for mannitol and 182°C for cocaine).

23. (bottom) The mannitol adulterant was removed from the sample shown above by taking the cocaine back to base and precipitating the cocaine hydrochloride from acetone.

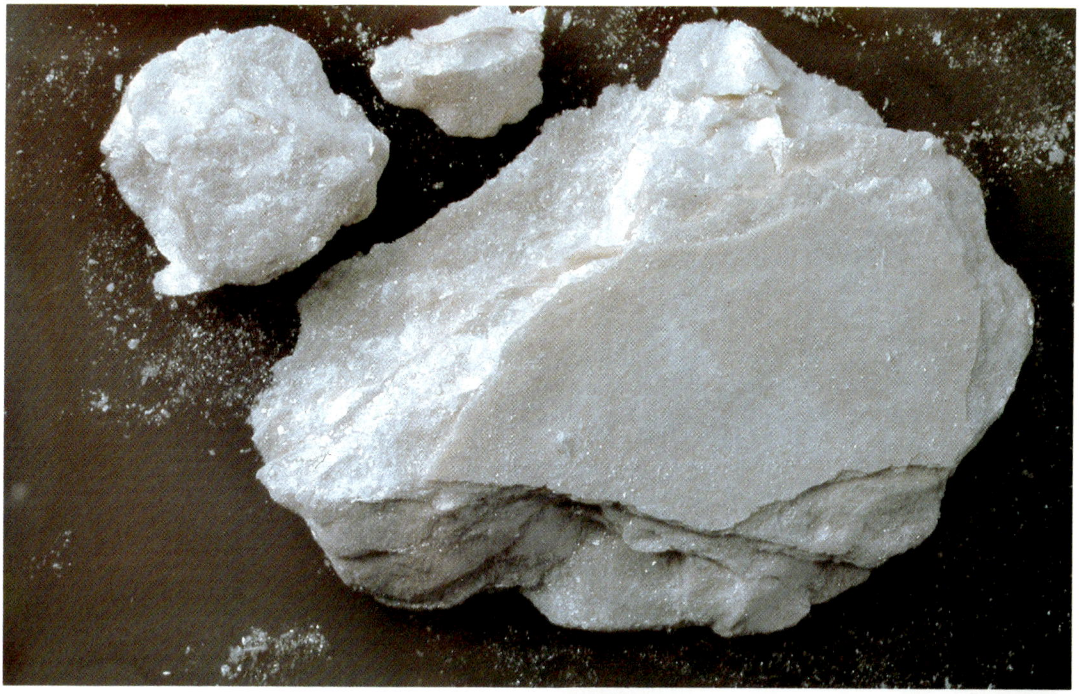

24. (above) **Cocaine pearl recovered from "supersoil," a highly contaminated disaster resembling dirt.**
25. (right) **Cocaine "crinkles" formed by fluted filter paper.**
26. (lower right) **Detail of cocaine shown in color plate 11.**

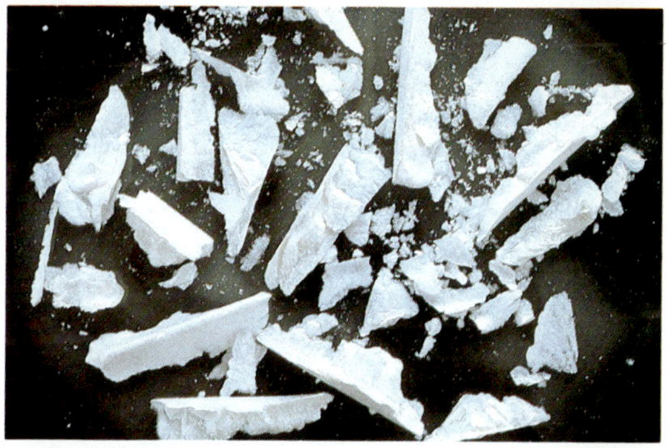

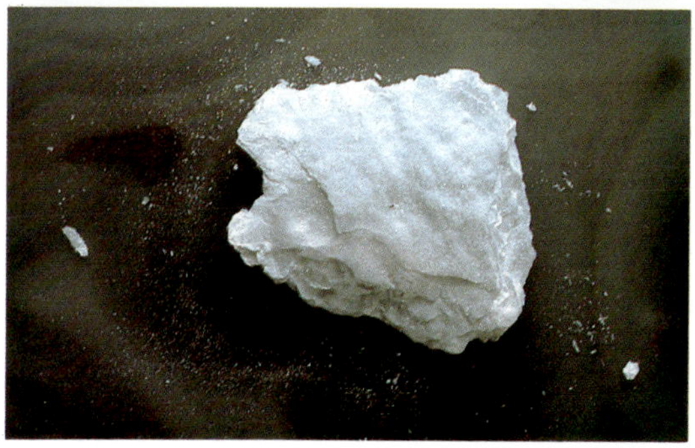

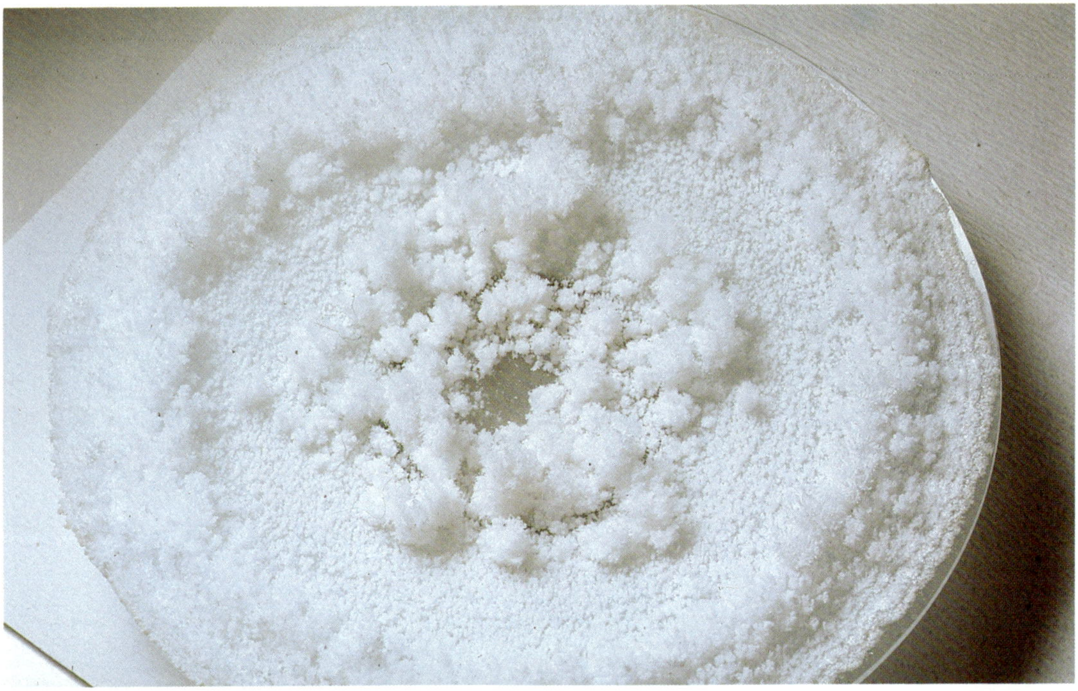

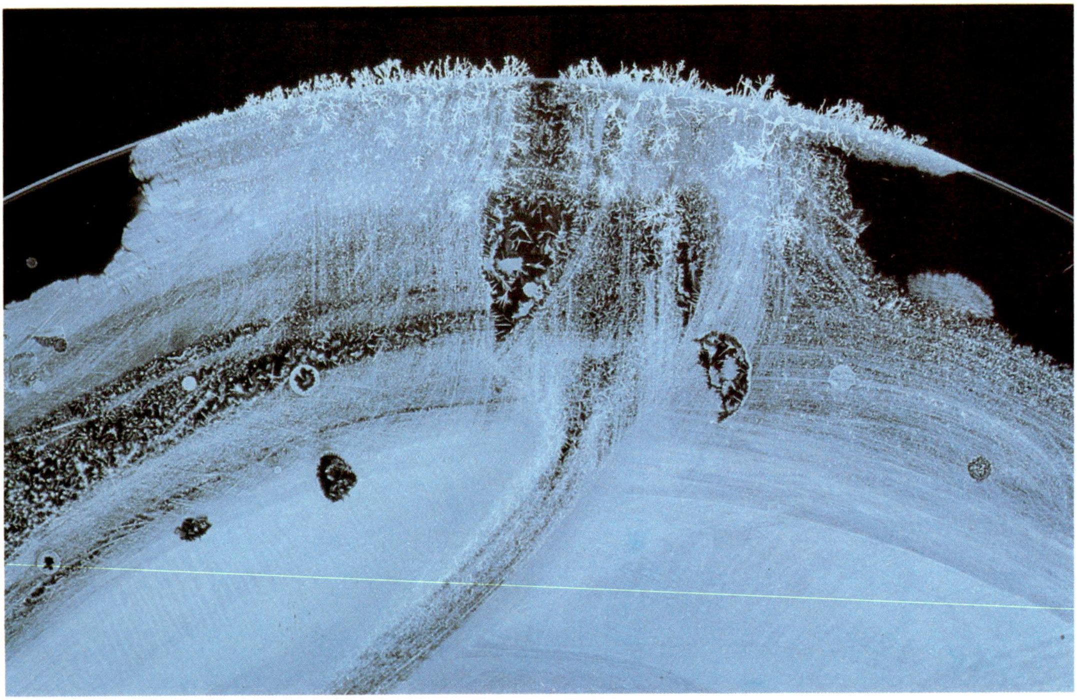

27. (top) This 14.5-gram cocaine base crystal formation in the 15-inch watchglass collapsed like a souffle shortly after the picture was taken. The base in photos was crystallized out of petroleum ether.
28. (bottom) "Cocaine base snow storm" on the edge of a watchglass.

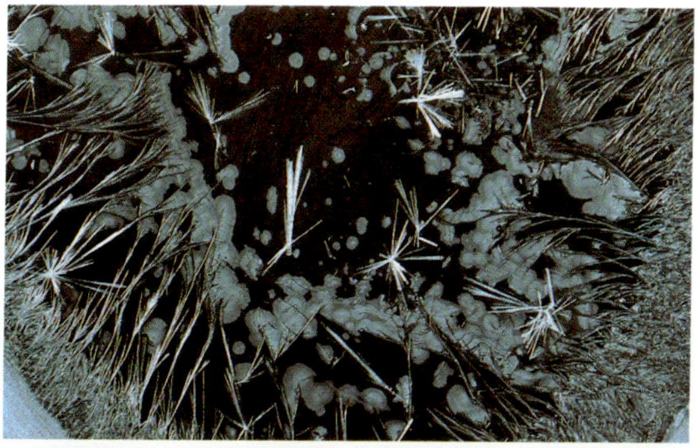

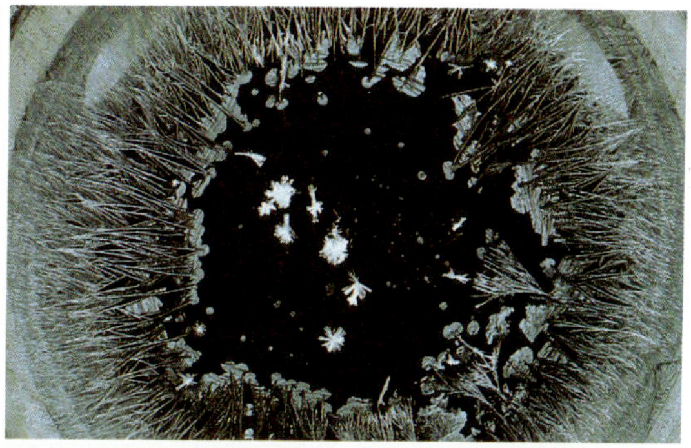

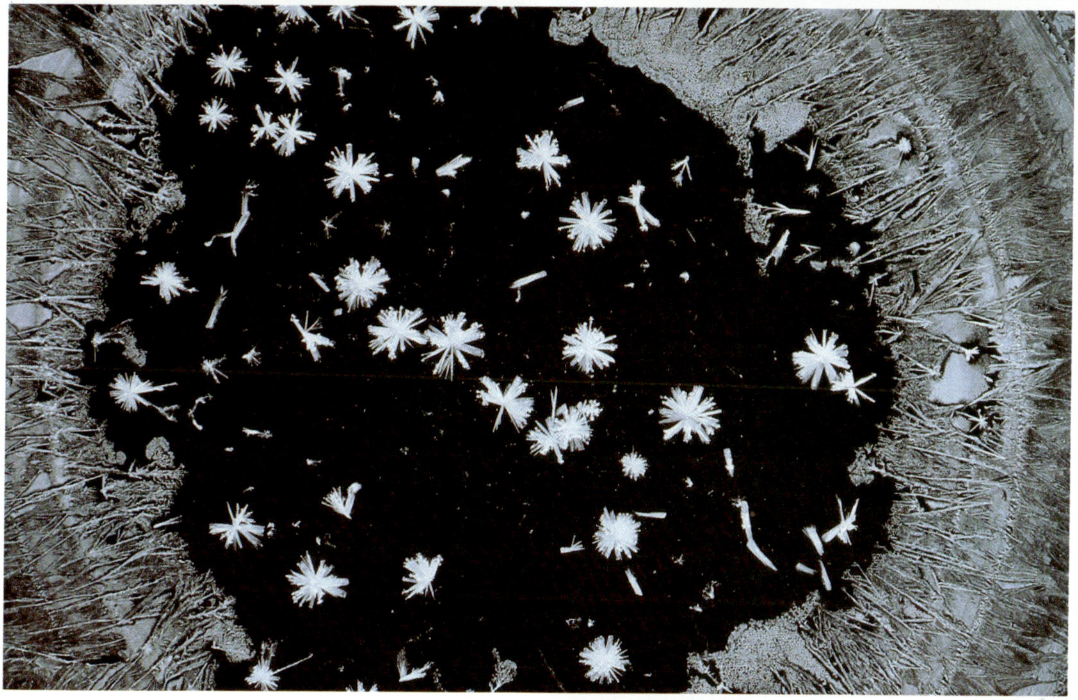

29., 30., & 31 (above) **Large crystals of cocaine base formed by slow evaporation of a dilute solution. The blue and gray areas contain oily impurities.**
32. (at right) **Residue from a "freebase" pipe rinsed out with petroleum ether.**

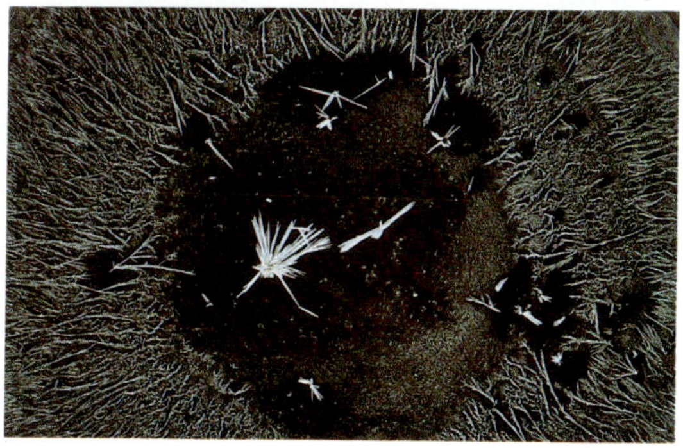

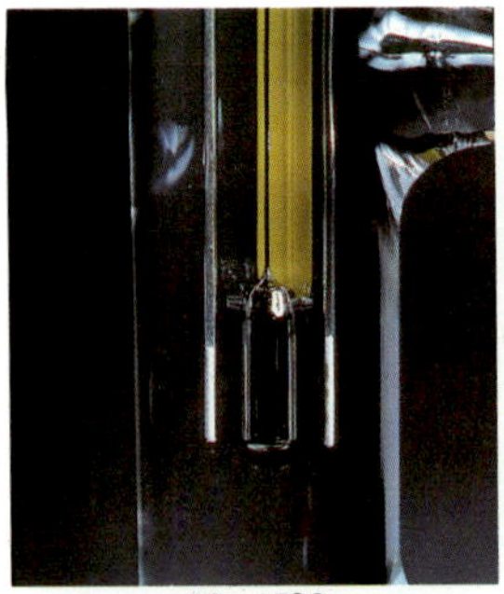

33. 15°C

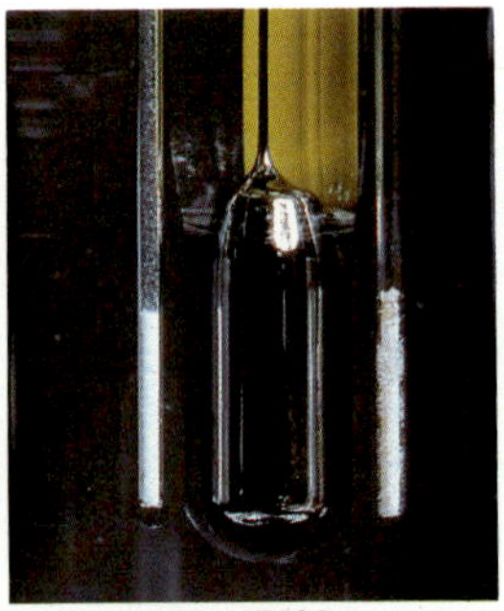

34. 170°C

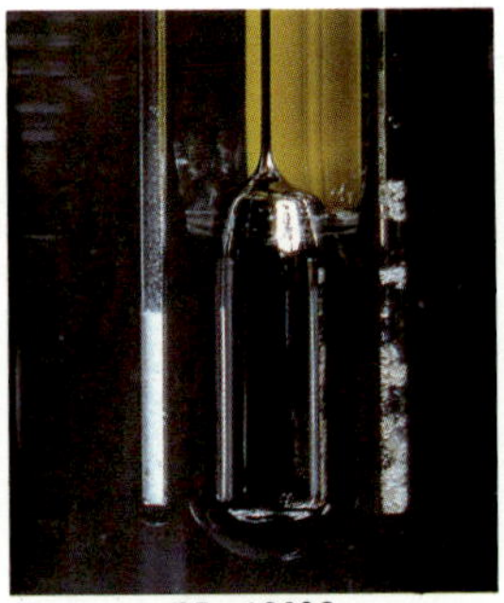

35. 180°C

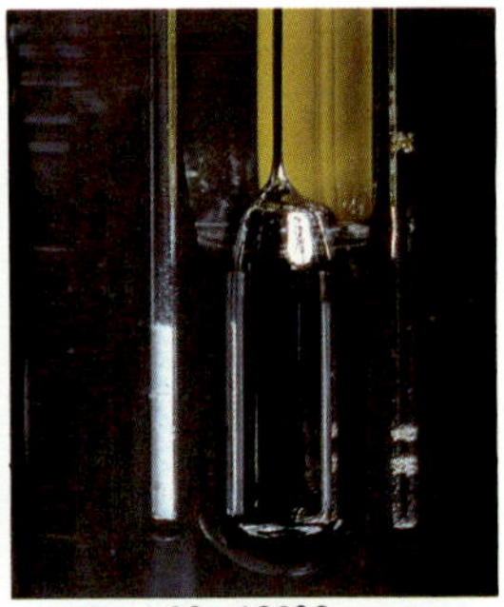

36. 182°C

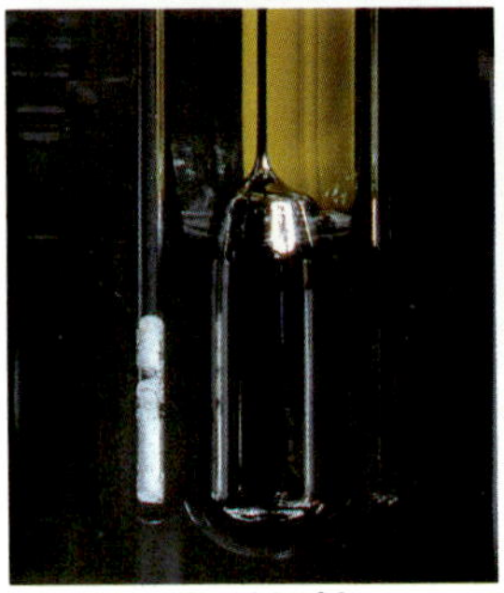

37. 186.5°C

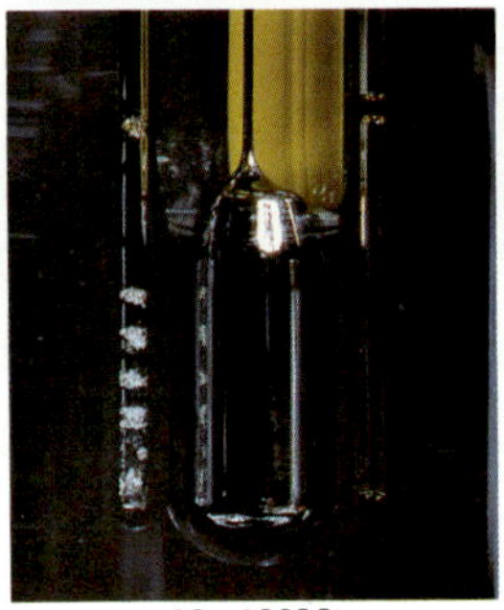

38. 188°C

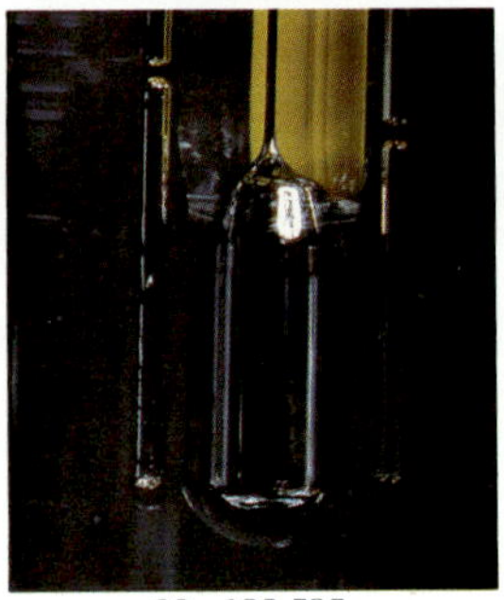

39. 188.5°C

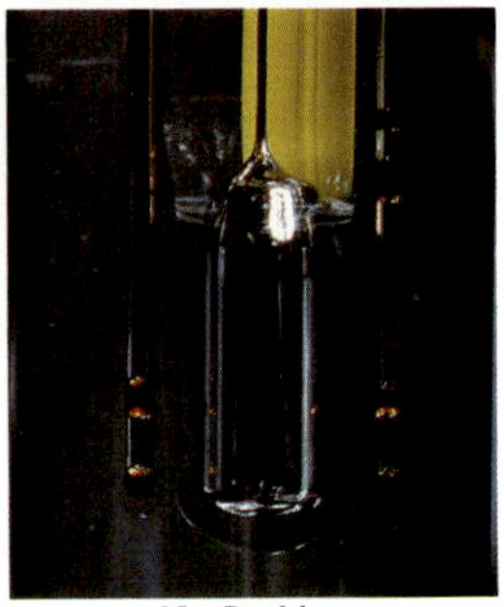

40. Residue

MELTING POINT TESTS

The photos on these two pages demonstrate results of melting point tests. Cocaine hydrochloride and adulterated samples are shown in capillary tubes at right and left of thermometer bulb in each photo. Temperature of sample shown is given below each photo. (For set-up of the melting point test, see black-and-white photos on pages 105, 108 and 109.)

33.-40. The series of photos above shows the melting of highly-refined illicit cocaine hydrochloride "BOOK STANDARD" in the capillary tube at the left of the thermometer bulb and "BOLIVIAN ROCK" in the capillary at the right of the bulb. The "Bolivian rock" started melting at about 170°C and finished at about 182°C; in contrast, the "book standard" had a sharp melting point 186.5°-188.0°C. This "Bolivian rock" was considered by consumers to be a high-quality product, so the melting point test is a sensitive indicator of impurities.

41.-48. (opposite page, top two rows) In left-hand capillary, cocaine hydrochloride cut with 25% MANNITOL starts melting at about 160°C and is finished at about 180°C. In the right-hand capillary, cocaine cut with 25% LACTOSE starts melting about 170°C and finishes about 182°C. In both cases, the residue after melting is a darker brown than that produced by cocaine alone; however, the lactose residue is much darker than that of mannitol.

49.-56. (opposite page, bottom two rows) In right-hand capillary tube, sample containing a 50% cut of MANNITOL, LACTOSE, and SPEED started melting below 120°C and was almost gone by 150°C. Sample in left-hand capillary, containing INOSITOL, started melting at about 180°C and finished about 187°C—a few particles remained at 187°C. The mannitol, lactose, and speed sample produced a dark residue at a temperature of 180°C; the inositol left a lighter residue (above 190°C).

SUMMARY OF MELTING POINT TESTS

Only the "book standard" purified illicit cocaine hydrochloride gave a sharp, high melting point—within a 1.5-degree range (186.5-188.0°C). Adulteration by 25% lowered the melting point and produced a wide range of melting—a spread of at least 10 degrees. With a 50% cut of mannitol, lactose, and speed, melting point started at about 120°C and finished at about 160°C—a 40 degree range.

The "Bolivian rock" and inositol-cut sample had similar melting point tests, so while the melting point will tell if a sample is fairly pure, a sample could fail the melting point test and still be of high quality. Another kind of test would be necessary to distinguish the "Bolivian rock" from the inositol cut. Inositol is one of several adulterants which require more than one test for detection.

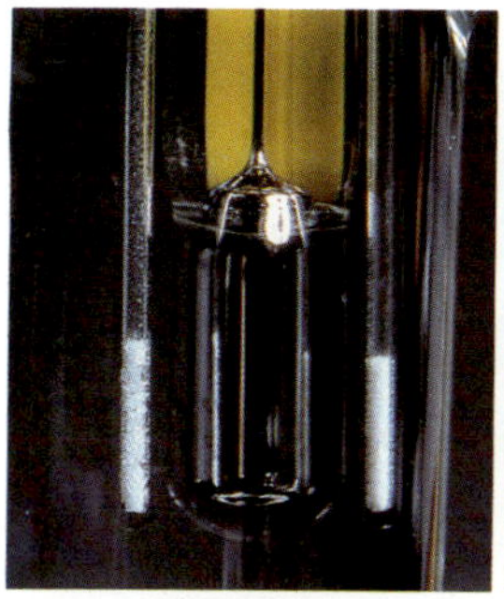

41. 160°C

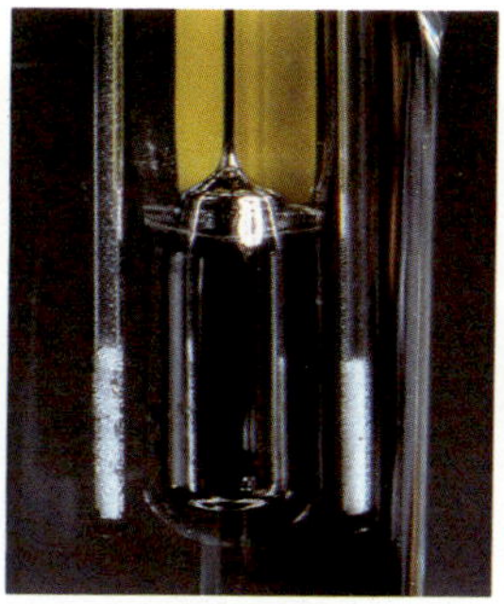

42. 165°C

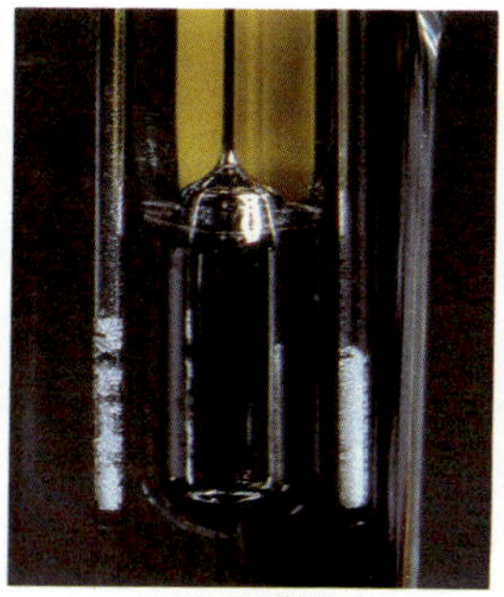

43. 169°C

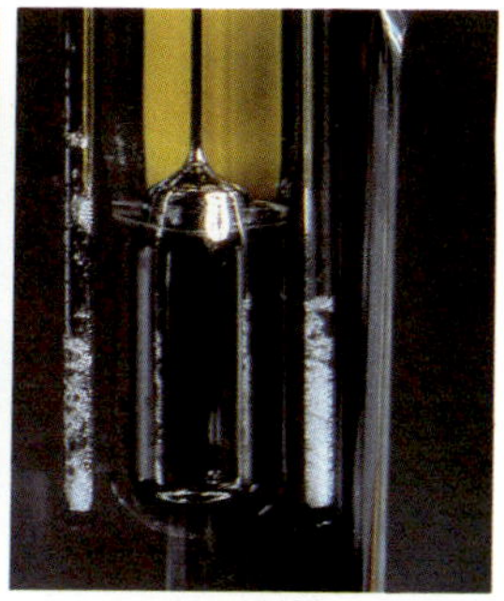

44. 172°C

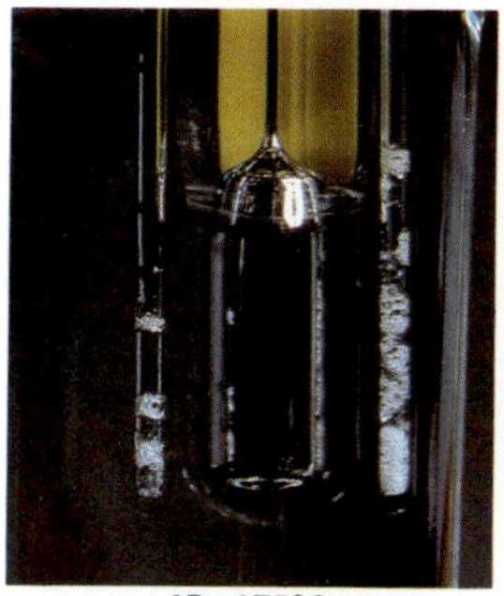

45. 175°C

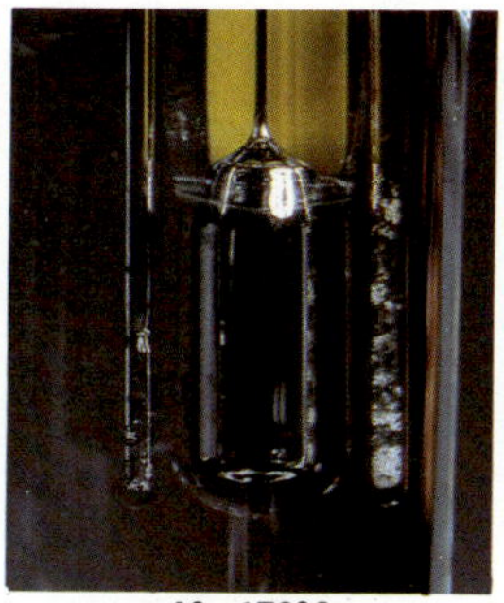

46. 178°C

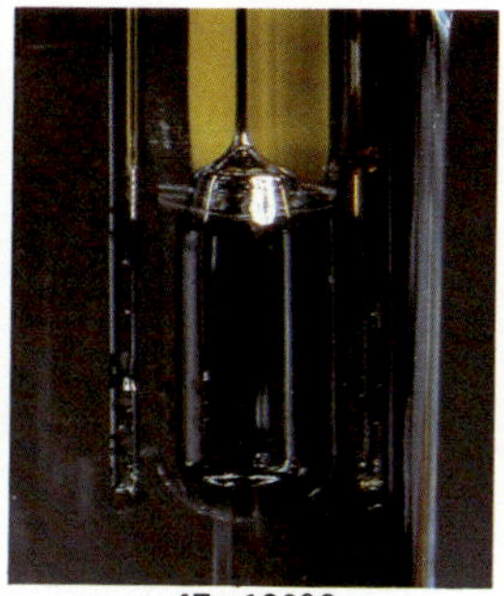

47. 182°C

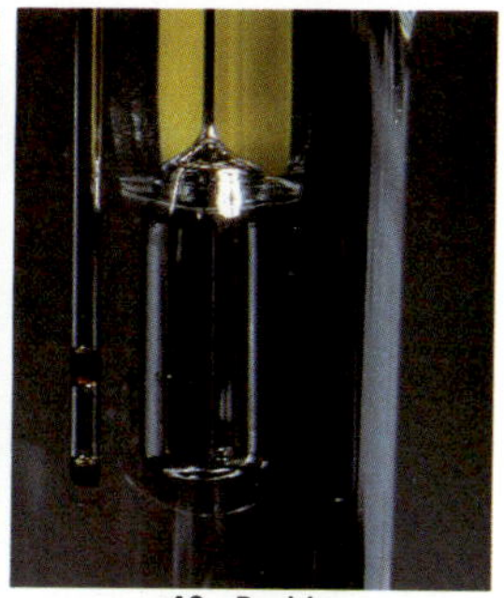

48. Residue

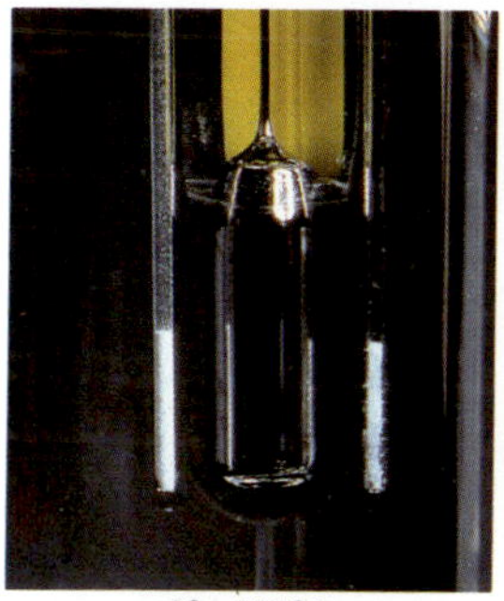

49. 115°C

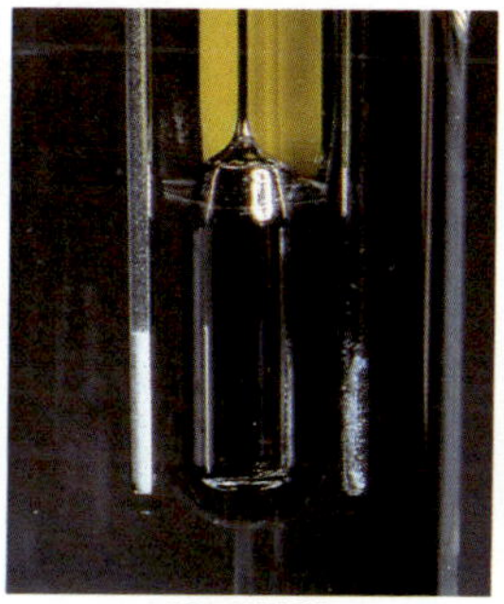

50. 125°C

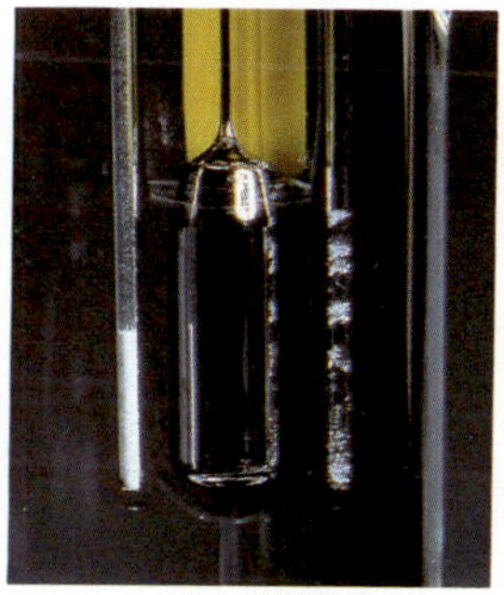

51. 139°C

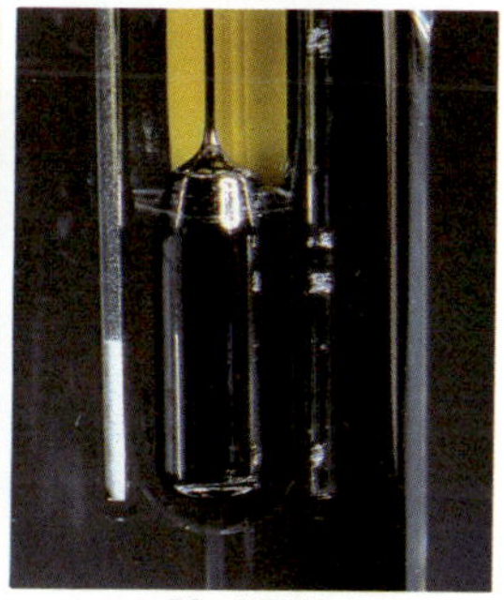

52. 150°C

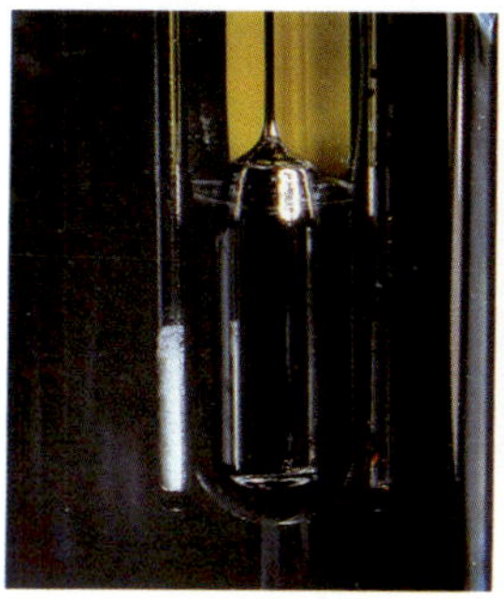

53. 181°C

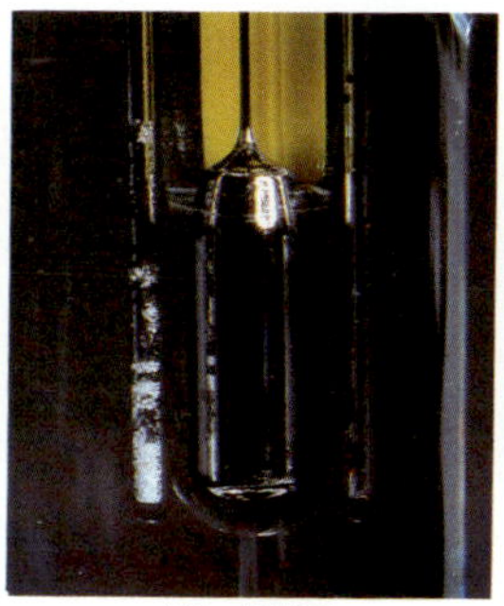

54. 185°C

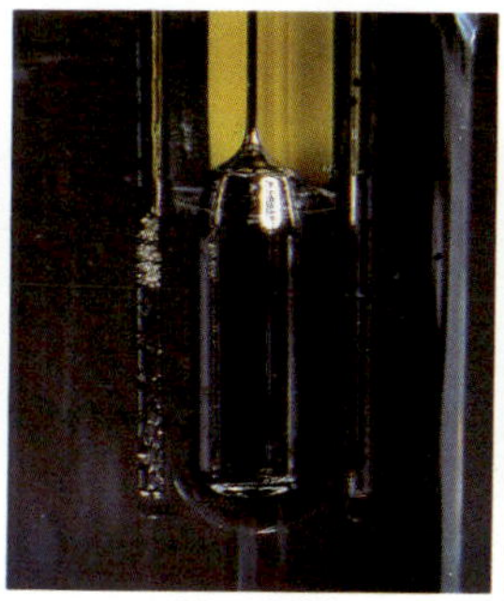

55. 187°C

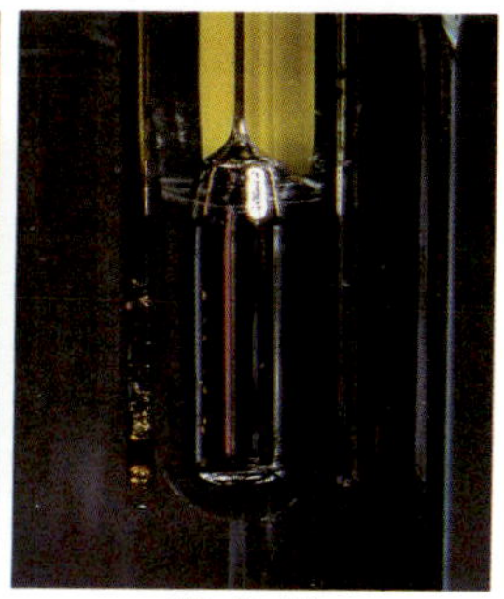

56. Residue

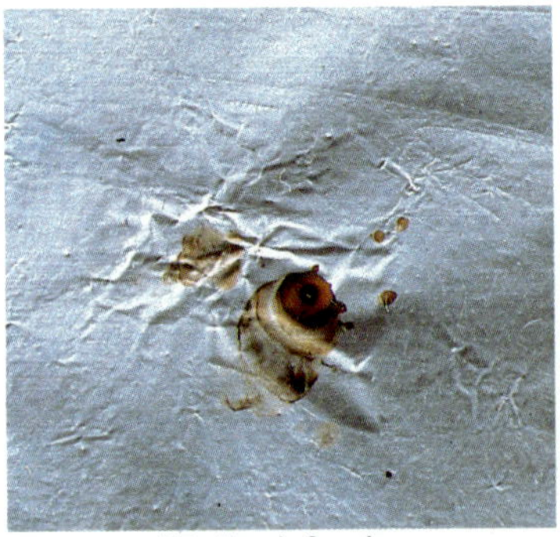

57. Merck Cocaine

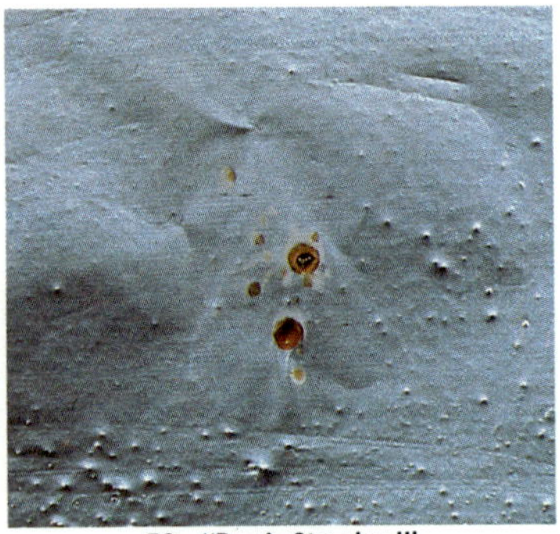

58. "Book Standard"

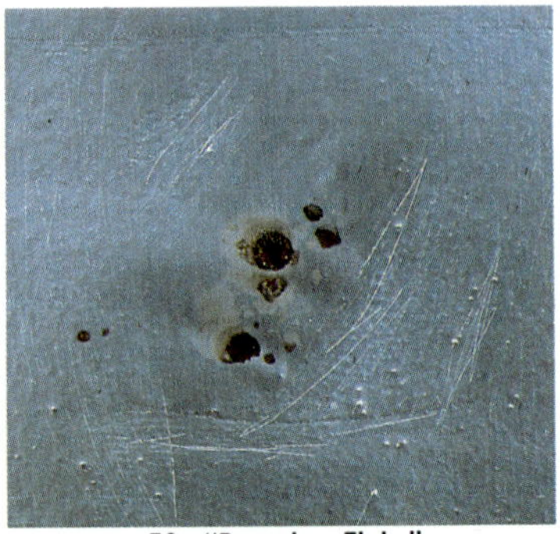

59. "Peruvian Flake"

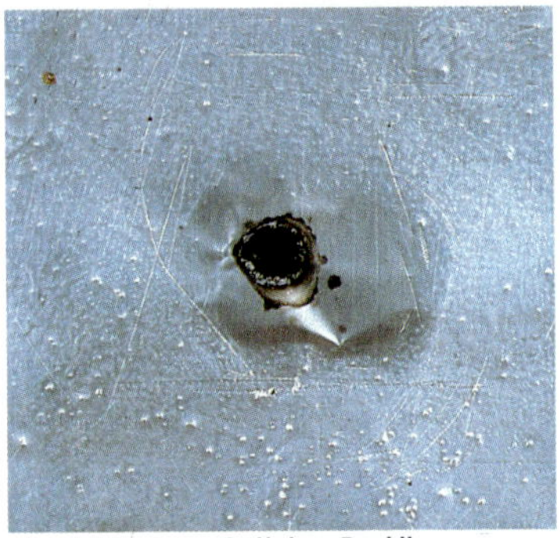

60. "Bolivian Rock"

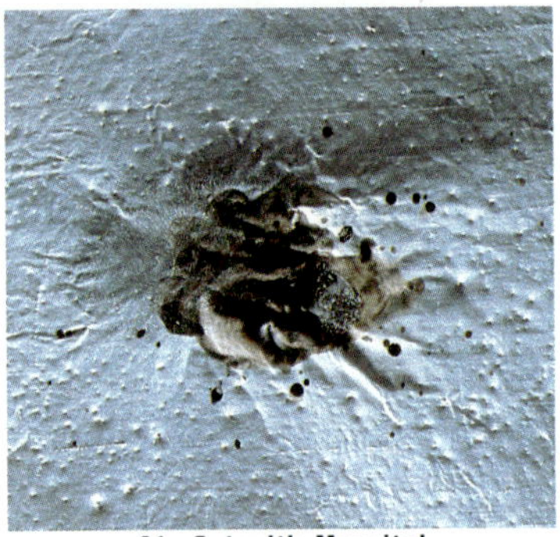

61. Cut with Mannitol

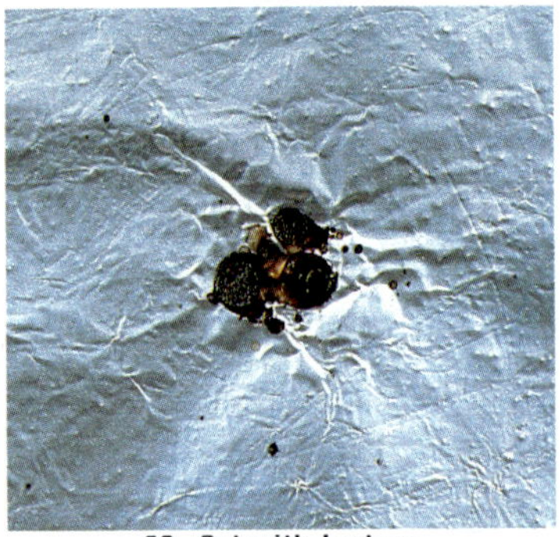

62. Cut with Lactose

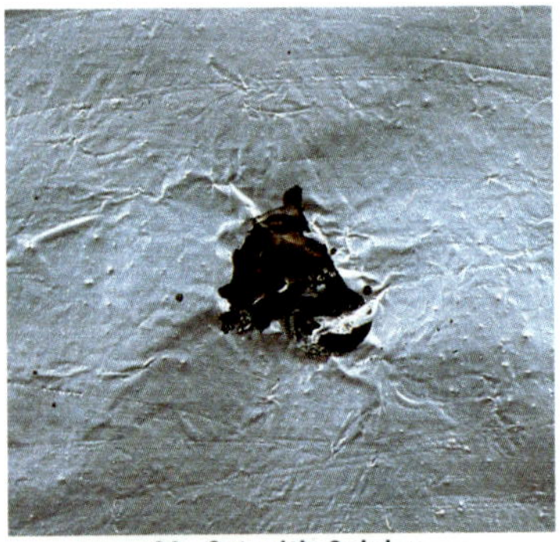

63. Cut with Quinine

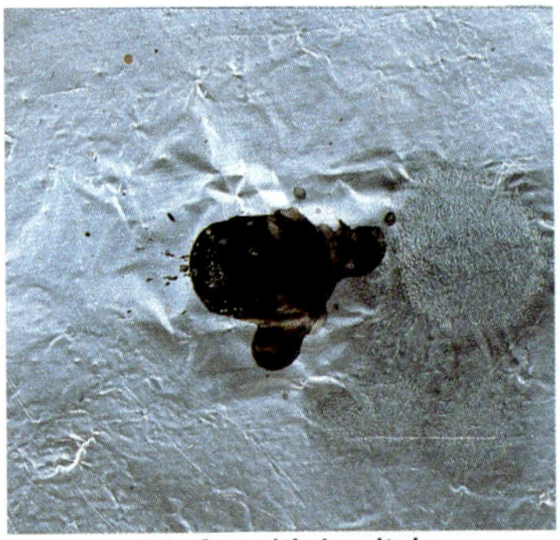

64. Cut with Inositol

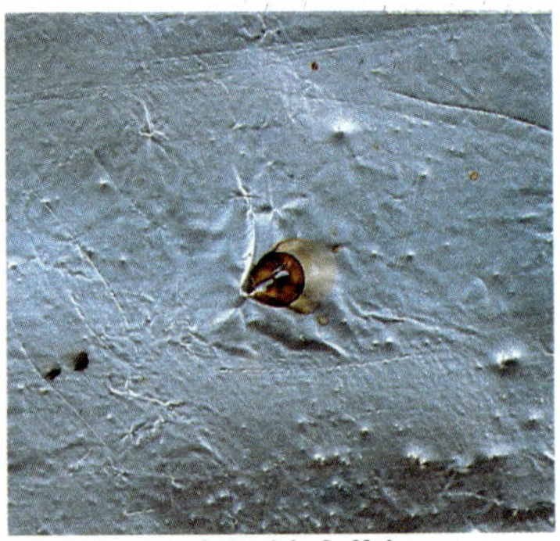

65. Cut with Caffeine

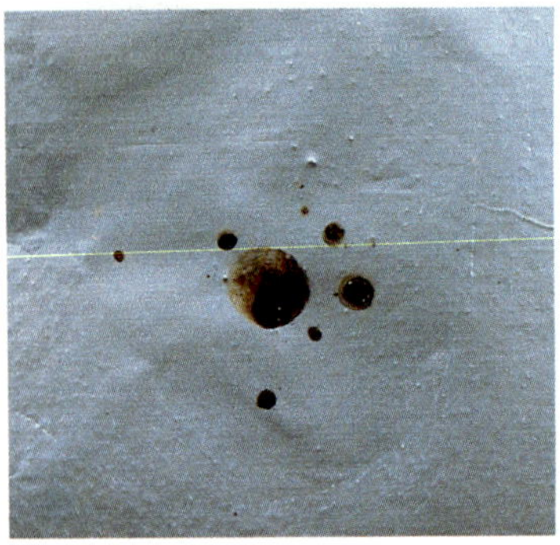

66. Cut with Lidocaine Hydrochloride

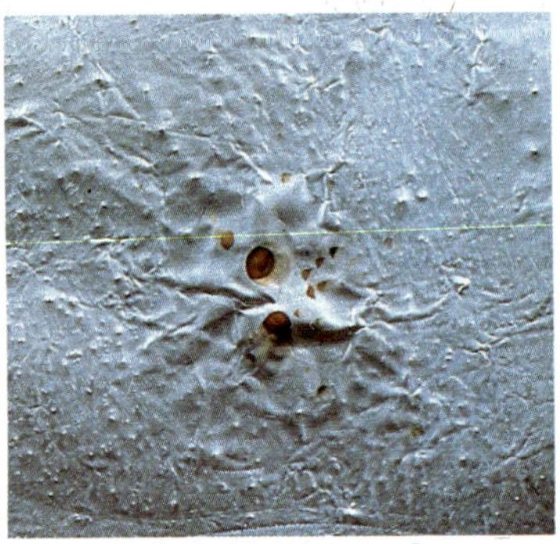

67. Cut with Lidocaine Base

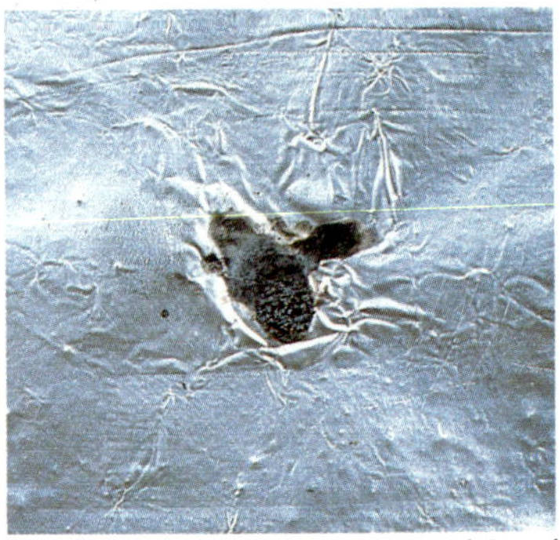

68. Cut with Mannitol, Lactose, and Speed

FOIL BURN TESTS

Foil burn tests as shown on the opposite page are done with about 10 milligrams of sample which is placed on aluminum foil and gently heated from below with a butane lighter. The residue is then examined. (For set-up of the foil burn test, see black-and-white photos on pages 102 and 103.)

57. (top row, left) **MERCK COCAINE: Even pharmaceutically pure cocaine leaves a small orange-brown residue.**

58. (top row, middle) **HIGHLY-REFINED ILLICIT COCAINE (the "Book standard") leaves a residue similar to that of pharmaceutical cocaine. The trace amounts of impurities account for the slightly darker color.**

59. (top row, right) **"PERUVIAN FLAKE": Although the sample was unadulterated, the presence of other alkaloids and impurities produces a darker brown residue than that shown in color plates 57 and 58.**

60. (second row, left) **"BOLIVIAN ROCK": While the cocaine content of "Bolivian rock" is usually higher than that of Peruvian, this sample was not well refined, and the impurities leave an almost black residue.**

In all the remaining tests, the "Book standard" cocaine was cut with different adulterants so that the sample used was 25% adulterant and 75% purified cocaine hydrochloride. For the test in the last color plate shown here, more adulterants were added so that the final sample contained 50% adulterants. In each instance (except the lidocaine hydrochloride and cocaine in color plate 66), the cocaine and cuts were mixed by screening them together.

61. (second row, middle) **COCAINE AND MANNITOL: Compared to color plate 58 (top row, middle), the added mannitol causes a black residue.**

62. (second row, right) **COCAINE AND LACTOSE: Here a black, charcoal-like residue is seen. The burning sample has a caramel consistency, and the smoke has the odor of burnt sugar.**

63. (third row, left) **COCAINE AND QUININE: When quinine is present, the residue is very pronounced, similar to a spot of dry India ink.**

64. (third row, middle) **COCAINE AND INOSITOL: This reacts much like the mannitol (second row, middle), but more burning is observed, and the residue is charcoal-like in appearance.**

65. (third row, right) **COCAINE AND CAFFEINE: The reaction of caffeine is so similiar to that of the "Book standard" cocaine (top row, middle) that this adulterant cannot be detected with the foil burn test.**

66. (bottom row, left) **COCAINE AND LIDOCAINE HYDROCHLORIDE: The residue here is slightly darker than "Book standard" (top row, middle), but shows no charcoal-like spot as in color plates 62 and 64. Detecting lidocaine with this test is virtually impossible.**

67. (bottom row, middle) **COCAINE AND LIDOCAINE BASE: When lidocaine base is the cut, the residue is almost identical to the "Book standard" cocaine.**

68. (bottom row, right) **COCAINE AND MANNITOL, LACTOSE, AND SPEED: This "street" cocaine has been cut a number of times; each time it is cut, it is more likely to fail the foil burn test.**

SUMMARY OF FOIL BURN TESTS

The foil burn test alone shows little conclusively. High-quality unrefined "Bolivian rock" cocaine can leave a dark residue, while cocaine cut with lidocaine or caffeine leaves very little residue. When sugar or quinine cuts are present, however, they always leave a dark residue. When combined with the results of other tests, information derived from foil burn tests can lead to more specific conclusions.

Chapter Seven

Purification

It would greatly simplify matters if illicit cocaine were sold with an accurate list of its contents. Since this is not the case, intuitive judgments must be made as to the quality of the cocaine and the nature of the adulterants which are present. In order to be effective, consumer oriented purification techniques must be general enough to apply under a wide range of circumstances. These procedures are not used to make cocaine; they are used to remove adulterants and impurities from cocaine that has already been made.

Since economics is always a prime factor in applying purification techniques, one point should be made clear. The cost of cocaine is dictated by the amount of it which is present in the original purchase (provided that none is lost in the purification process). If a gram costs $100 and is only 50% cocaine, the actual cost of the cocaine is $200 per gram. Consumers who use a purification method to remove adulterants frequently find the resulting purer cocaine too intense, and add an adulterant of their own choosing (much as someone would take hard liquor with soda or water) or simply use much less. The real difference between snorting one gram of 50% cocaine or one half gram of pure lies in the other 50%, the contents of which can clog the nose, numb the brain, stiffen the muscles, or just do nothing.

The Acetone Wash

When cocaine burns the nose, the problem may be that it has not been washed properly at the end of the manufacturing process. Most of the illicit cocaine consumed in the United States comes complete with excess hydrochloric acid and an overabundance of oily organic material like hygrine. This extra acid was added in order to speed up the crystallization process and force the oil out of an ether solution with the cocaine. The oil, which may make up as much as 50% of the hydrochloride weight, might otherwise remain in the ether. Once the crystallization is complete, the cocaine, plus oils, plus excess acid are collected by filtration. The ether will pass through the filter and the solids will remain. Much of the extra acid and some of the impurities could be removed at this point if fresh solvent was poured over the cocaine and allowed to pass through the filter; this is called a *wash.* Since most suppliers of illicit cocaine desire a maximum yield, the wash is often deleted. To further complicate matters, the filtered cocaine is rarely dried completely. This adds a small amount of weight in the form of solvent residue.

The dangers of snorting cocaine which contains even small amounts of hydrochloric acid and/or ether residue should be quite obvious. These chemicals will not only sting the nose on contact but may well cause deterioration of the nasal membrane. In addition, they are likely to cause headaches with repeated use. Hygrine acts as a local irritant on the nasal membranes. While this is partially due to the acid which it contains, hygrine is poorly absorbed in the nose and will remain long after the cocaine has dissolved. If the nose is not properly cleaned, membrane damage may be the result.

It is unnecessary for the consumer to subject himself to this kind of humiliation. The cure is as simple as the cause. All that is necessary to correct the problem is to

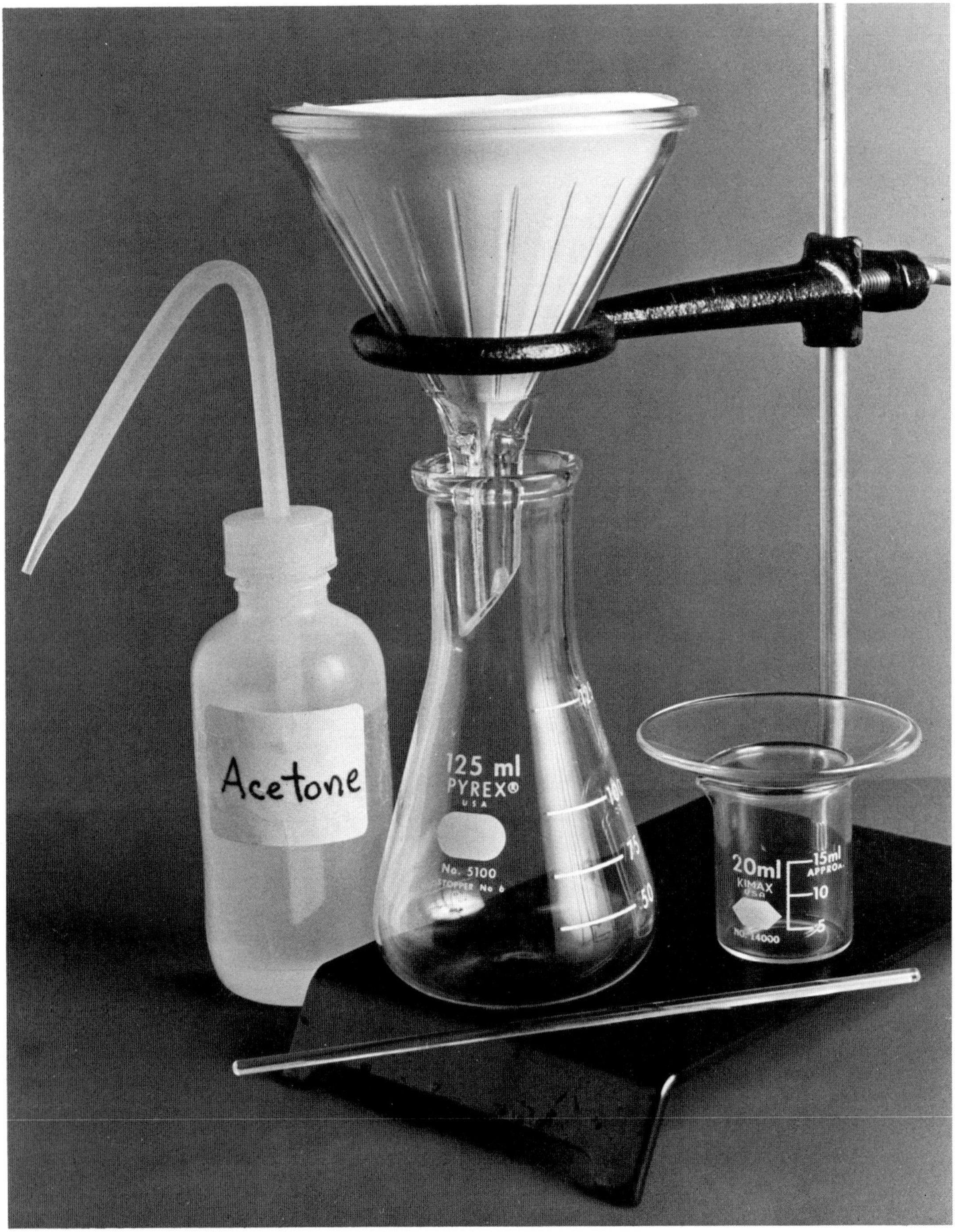

96. The equipment used for the acetone wash includes: acetone in a plastic wash bottle, a 125ml Erlenmeyer flask, a ribbed funnel with a medium-speed filter paper, a 20ml beaker with a watch-glass cover, a glass stirring rod, a lab stand.

complete those parts of the process which were omitted. Since the cocaine did not receive a final wash, it is put back in solvent so that this simple procedure can be properly performed.

The most efficient way to wash cocaine (HCl) is by decantation. This technique is routinely used to separate a fine wine from any sediment which it may contain. In washing cocaine the solvent in which the cocaine was crystallized is poured off. This solution is called the mother liquor. After decanting the mother liquor, fresh solvent is added to the cocaine to remove more of the impurities and excess acid. The fresh solvent and cocaine are swirled together and allowed to stand until the cocaine has settled to the bottom. The solvent on top may then be decanted also. Each time this procedure is done, the cocaine is washed.

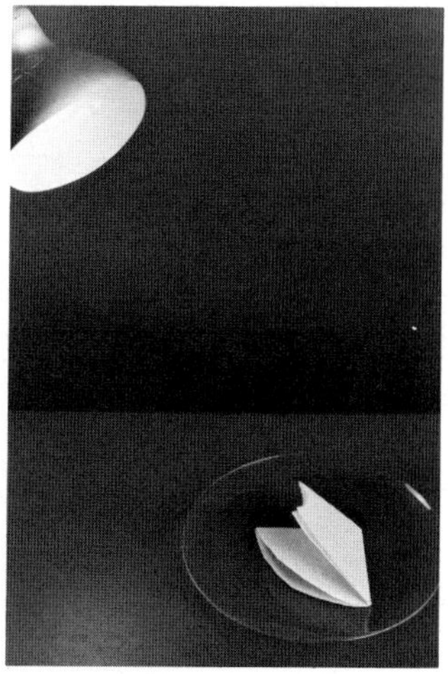

97. The filter paper is heated just before use to remove moisture.

In the case of cocaine which has been crystallized but not washed, the mother liquor has already been removed. The wash procedure must begin by placing the cocaine in a beaker and covering it with fresh solvent. A small stirring rod is used to break up pieces so that the insoluble material (the cocaine) is of an even consistency. The entire contents of the beaker are swirled and covered with a watchglass. In a few minutes, the cocaine will settle to the bottom and the solvent with its soluble impurities will be on top. When all the solid particles have settled to the bottom, the solvent is decanted through a filter and collected in a separate container. Any cocaine which is accidentally poured off with the solvent will remain in the filter. The cocaine which remained in the beaker is covered with fresh solvent, swirled, and the entire contents poured into the filter. Once all the solvent has passed through the filter, a small portion of fresh solvent is poured over the cocaine and allowed to pass through the filter. Any soluble impurities which may have been trapped at the bottom of the filter cone will be the first to pass through the filter when this is done.

This type of filtration is called gravity filtration. It is based on the same principle which is used to filter coffee the "Melitta way." When a solid is separated from a liquid

(Continued on page 153)

WARNING!

Some of the procedures documented, especially those involving volatile solvents or concentrated acids and alkalis may be extremely hazardous. The reader is cautioned not to perform any of these procedures. The procedures described should only be performed under laboratory conditions by professional chemists operating under the authority of the proper government regulatory agencies.

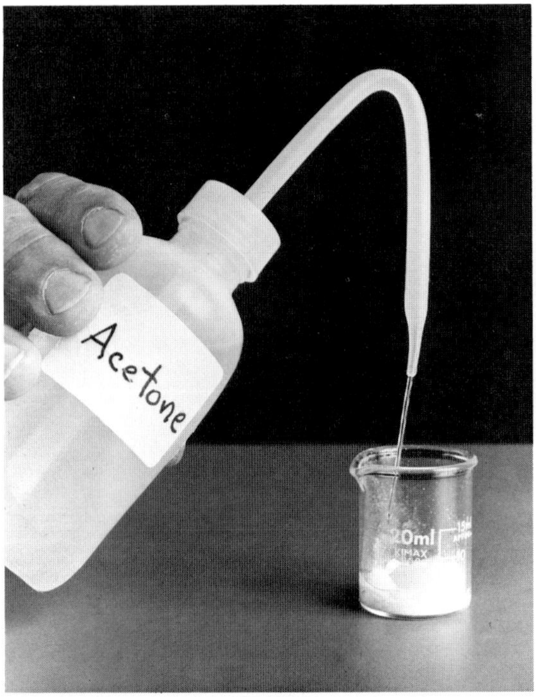

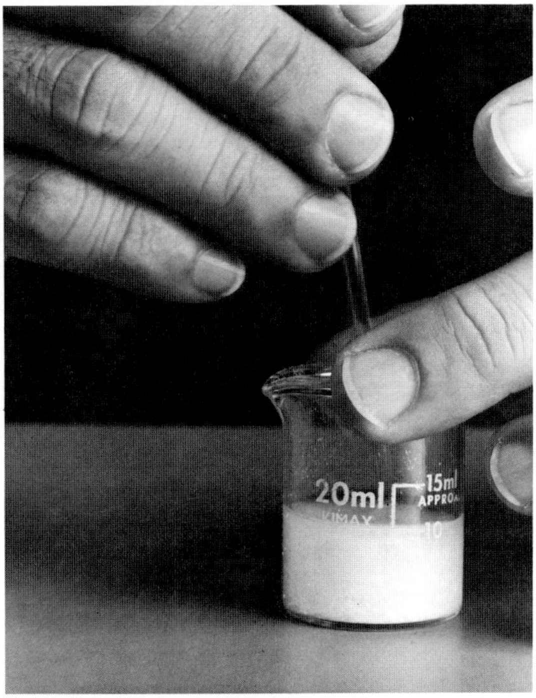

top:

98. Ten milliliters of acetone is added to one gram of sample.

99. Acetone and sample are stirred for one to two minutes.

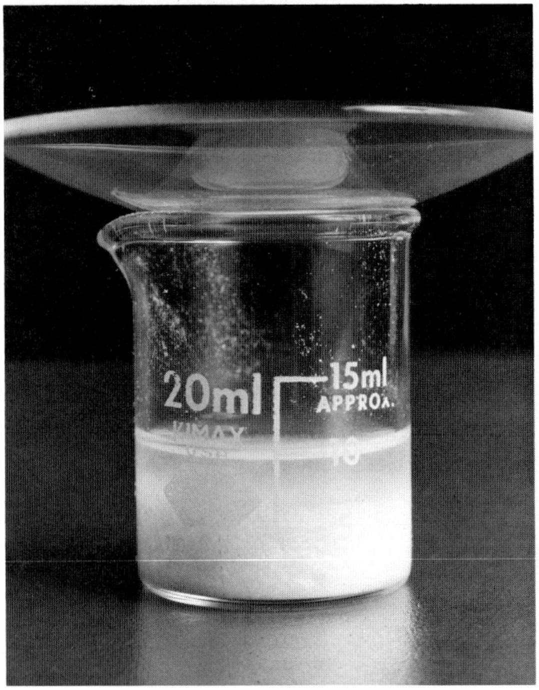

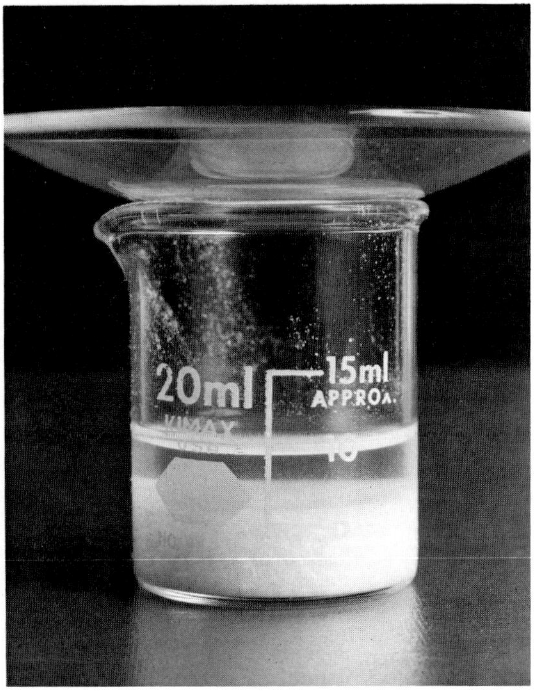

bottom:

100. Crystals are allowed to settle to the bottom. The watchglass prevents dirt from falling into beaker.

101. When crystals have settled, acetone above is clear.

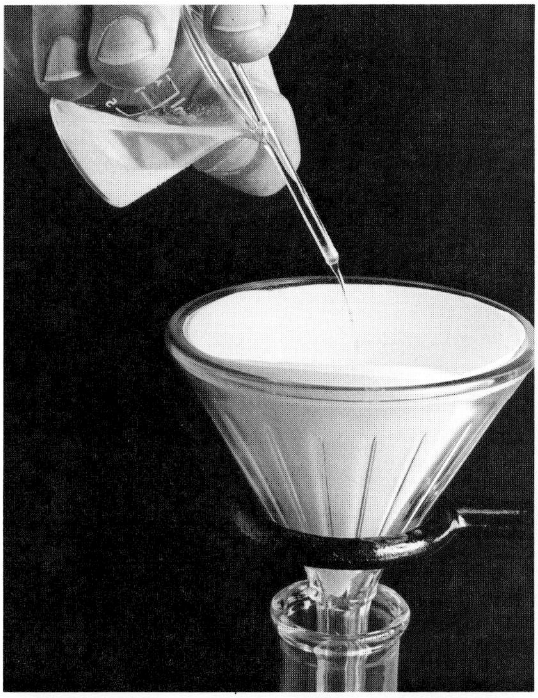

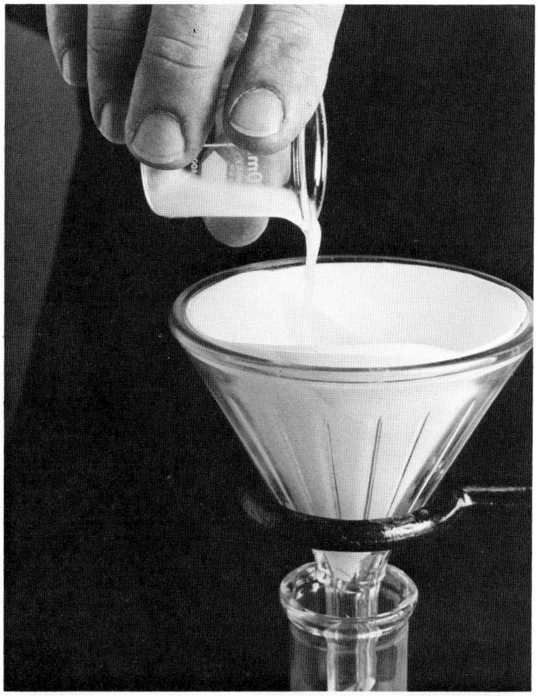

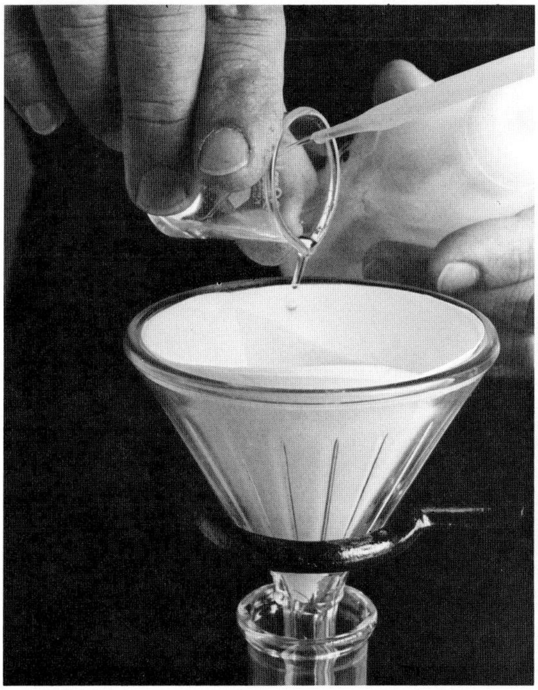

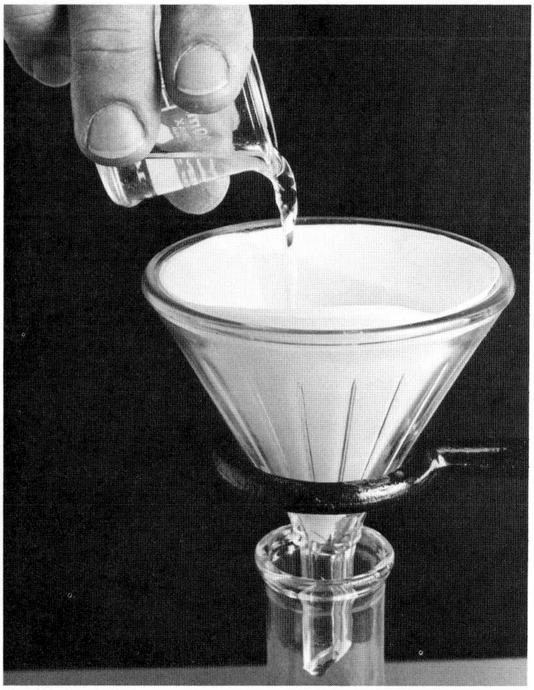

top:

102. Acetone is decanted off the crystals through filter and into flask. Stirring rod guides the liquid and prevents spills.
103. Steps in photos 98 and 99 (p. 150) are repeated and the entire contents are poured into the center of the filter.

bottom:

104. The beaker is rinsed with acetone to remove traces of sample.
105. After all the acetone has passed through, an additional 10ml of fresh acetone is poured over the sample.

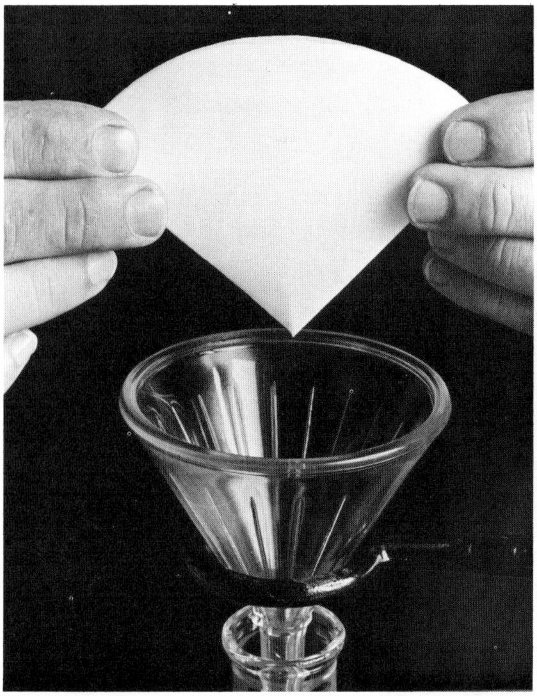
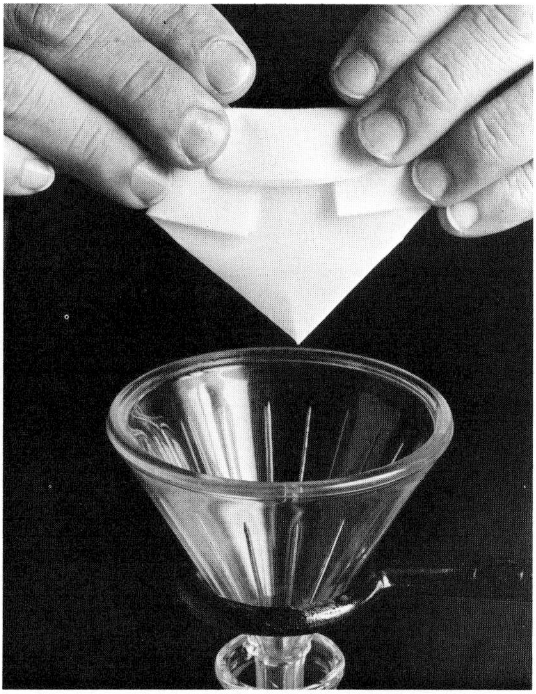
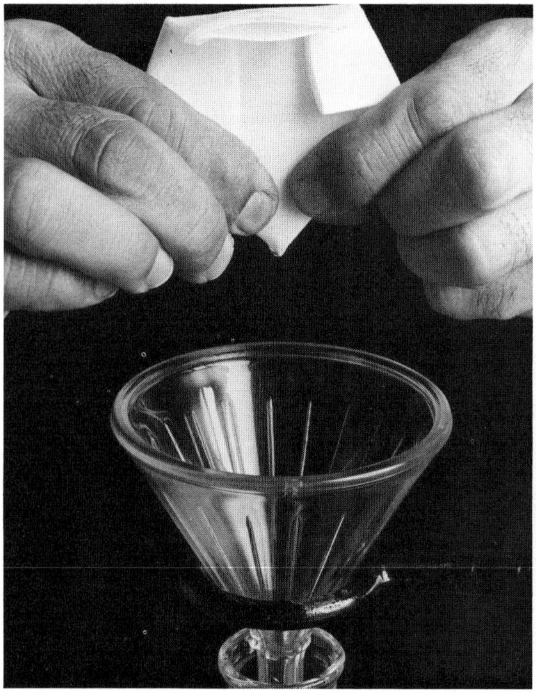
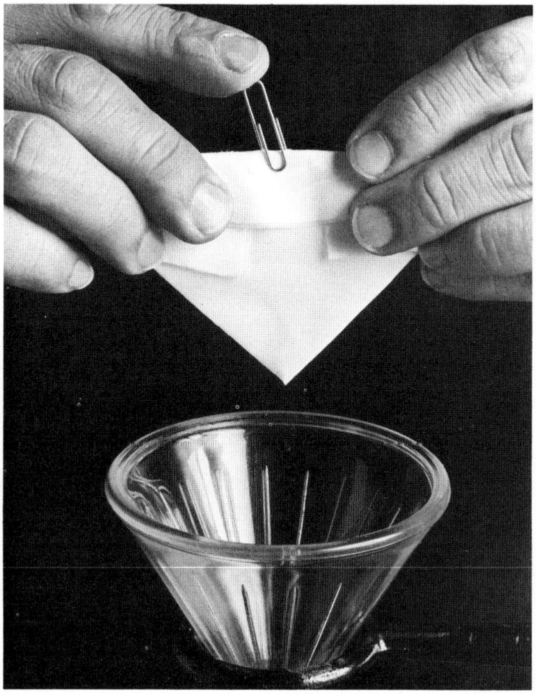

top:

106. When all the acetone has passed through, the filter cone is removed from the funnel.
107. Then it is folded in at sides, and lastly, down at top.

bottom:

108. The last drop of acetone is squeezed out.
109. A paper clip secures the folds. The folded filter with contents is then placed under a heat lamp to dry.

(Continued from page 149)

by gravity filtration, there will always be traces of solvent which remain in the solid. These are removed by evaporation. To facilitate this, the filter cone containing the solid material is pressed between the hands in a downward motion so that most of the remaining solvent will be forced out the bottom. The trace of solvent which remains is evaporated when the filter cone, complete with cocaine, is placed under a heat lamp to dry. The filter paper acts as a protective shell, preventing the cocaine from being exposed directly to the heat lamp.

The choice of solvent is a critical one which must satisfy certain criteria. Most important of these is that the solvent dissolve the impurities without dissolving the cocaine. Second, it must evaporate at a temperature lower than that which would melt the cocaine, and it should leave no residue once evaporated.

One solvent which meets all of these criteria is acetone. Contrary to cocaine mythology, acetone is an excellent solvent which leaves 0.001% residue after evaporation. Cocaine hydrochloride is almost totally insoluble in acetone, but hydrochloric acid will totally dissolve. Hygrine hydrochloride and other organic impurities are partially soluble in acetone. The base forms of most drugs used to adulterate cocaine are very soluble in acetone. Acetone is extremely flammable but will not form explosive peroxides as does anhydrous diethyl ether. It is the peroxides which can simply explode when dried and are probably the cause of frequently reported and rumored "underground" laboratory fires.* Acetone is sold in several grades which vary in purity. It is important that the acetone be "chemically pure," that is, free from alcohol and water, both of which will dissolve cocaine.

Aside from purifying the cocaine, the acetone wash may significantly improve its aesthetics. It is often the

---

* Some solvents mentioned here and many solvents used routinely in laboratories are toxic and/or flammable (possibly explosive). Working with them where ventilation is inadequate creates a LIFE THREATENING situation. Safe use of such solvents is a complex problem which professional laboratories have solved; any layman using such solvents is risking his life.

Cocaine Solubility—
In acidic and basic solutions

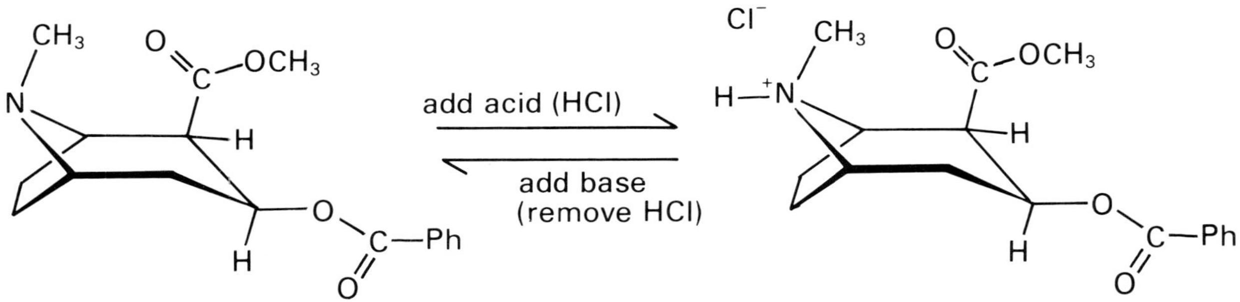

Cocaine

Base Form—(high pH)—
no electric charge,
soluble in organic solvents,
insoluble in water

Cocaine hydrochloride

Salt Form—(low pH)—
has electric charge,
soluble in water,
insoluble in organic solvents

Ph = 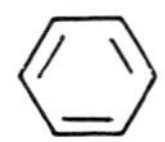

impurities which obscure cocaine's crystallinity.

The acetone wash will seldom if ever lower the quality of cocaine. However, it does have negative aspects which should also be understood. First, there is bound to be a weight loss, usually 8–12%, very little of which will be cocaine. Second, cocaine which is washed in acetone cannot be consumed for at least 48 hours after it is dry. The aging process is critical to the taste and smell of the cocaine as well as the health of the consumer. Aging is even more effective when the cocaine is screened to a fine powder, spread out on a non-porous surface, and dried under heat.

Finally, since the quality of the washed cocaine is likely to be much better than its predecessor, it is much easier to consume larger amounts in a shorter period of time. The negative effects of dirty cocaine often act as a deterrent to its use; when the dirt is removed, so is the deterrent.

As they say in Colombia, "The chef is everything." Their differing skills affect both the appearance and the head of the cocaine they produce. But the exact extent of their influence isn't always ascertainable. Obviously the hash slingers of the big commercial kitchens don't prepare the yellow rock or the pink flake, much less the silvery butterfly wings and iridescent mother-of-pearl featured by the great chefs. But there is no objective data on how, say, a chef's ability to alter the percentage and ratios of the noncocaine alkaloids remaining in the illicit product affect the high. And unless a great chef publishes his or her observations on the subject, we are not likely to learn how the different solvents—petroleum ether, benzene, alcohol, to name a few—affect the appearance.

Richard Ashley, *High Times*, 1979.

Crystallization

In this context, crystallization is a term used to refer to the process of converting cocaine base to cocaine hydrochloride. This requires technical skills which are similar to those used to convert cocaine hydrochloride to cocaine base. The major difference is that the hydrochloride form is usually the finished product which will be sold on the black market. Its aesthetic and technical qualities greatly influence the selling price and will be the subject of close examination. The base, on the other hand, is not the final product and therefore does not require the precision and sophistication necessary to produce a marketable item. It is a means to an end, and its aesthetic qualities are of little importance.

Base is made by dissolving cocaine hydrochloride in distilled water and slowly adding an alkali like ammonium hydroxide. This raises the pH of the solution sufficiently for the cocaine base to precipitate. When it has been determined that precipitation is complete, the base is separated from the water by filtration or extraction with petroleum ether.

The dry base is reconverted to the hydrochloride by dissolving it in ether or acetone, and adding hydrochloric acid. As the pH is lowered, the cocaine precipitates as cocaine hydrochloride crystals. When it has been determined that crystallization is complete, the crystals are separated from the solvents (mother liquor) by filtration.

This, at least, is the science which by laboratory standards involves relatively simple procedures. The art is another story, which to the present day has retained its secrecy. This mystique has given power to those who know its secrets—power over those who lack this understanding. For the cocaine connoisseur, there is no denying the aesthetic appeal and subsequent desire created by the look of iridescent flakes of cocaine which when fractured reveal layered caverns of mother-of-pearl cocaine. The testing kits are forgotten when the cocaine looks like cocaine, and people who could not afford dinner come out of the woodwork with sufficient cash to pay for dessert. They call it "the kind," a rare sight even among connoisseurs.

CRYSTALLIZATION OF COCAINE HYDROCHLORIDE:
Problems and Remedies

INDICATION	CAUSE	REMEDY
The base will not totally dissolve in acetone.	The base was improperly made or poorly washed. Some HCl remains.	The insoluble part is removed by filtration. It may then be redissolved in water and converted to base.
	The base may contain a non-acetone-soluble adulterant.	If insoluble in water, it is discarded.
The acid is added and no reaction occurs.	The chemicals are too cold; stirring is insufficient.	The chemicals are warmed to room temperature. The combined solution is reswirled until the reaction begins.
	Not enough acid was used to sufficiently lower the pH.	The pH is lowered by adding more acid.
The final hydrochloride weight is less than the base weight.	The base was not totally dry when dissolved in acetone and an incorrect weight was the result.	The base must be completely dry before crystallizing.
	The base contained an oily substance which did not precipitate with the cocaine.	The oil base is not cocaine and is allowed to remain in the mother liquor.

Even in cocaine producing countries the situation is much the same. High quality flake cocaine has become so rare that high ranking members of larger cocaine organizations often have their own chemist who makes special batches of "the kind" for themselves and a few close associates. While the science is readily available to anyone who can read, the art is only known to a select few.

The science of crystallization is chemistry. In order to control the technical and aesthetic qualities of cocaine, the artist must understand the factors which, when properly manipulated, will produce the look which is desired. As this applies to flake cocaine, the factors are the conditions during crystal growth and crystal drying.

Crystal Growth

The way that cocaine crystals grow is dependent on the characteristics of the base and the rate at which the pH is lowered. The more rapidly this change occurs, the smaller will be the resultant crystals. The slower the pH is changed, the larger the crystals. The artist seeks to avoid extreme changes whether they be slow or rapid. One gram may be crystallized in as little as 5 minutes or as long as 48 hours.

The majority of the great cooks agree that the best looking flake is made from crystals which were all precipitated at the same time and then allowed to grow in size over a period of hours. The resultant crystals are of equal size and consistency, and so is the flake. When crystallization is too rapid, the crystals, while homogenous in size and consistency, retain impurities which dull the sparkle necessary to make pearl. Crystals which grow too slowly are usually the result of improper mixing of the acid and the base. These larger crystals, while brilliant in appearance, are usually unequal in size. They tend to retain solvents which do not "go away" when dried, and, where trapped acid is involved, multiple problems can occur. These include lowered yields and extremely acidic cocaine which can damage the nasal passage when snorted.

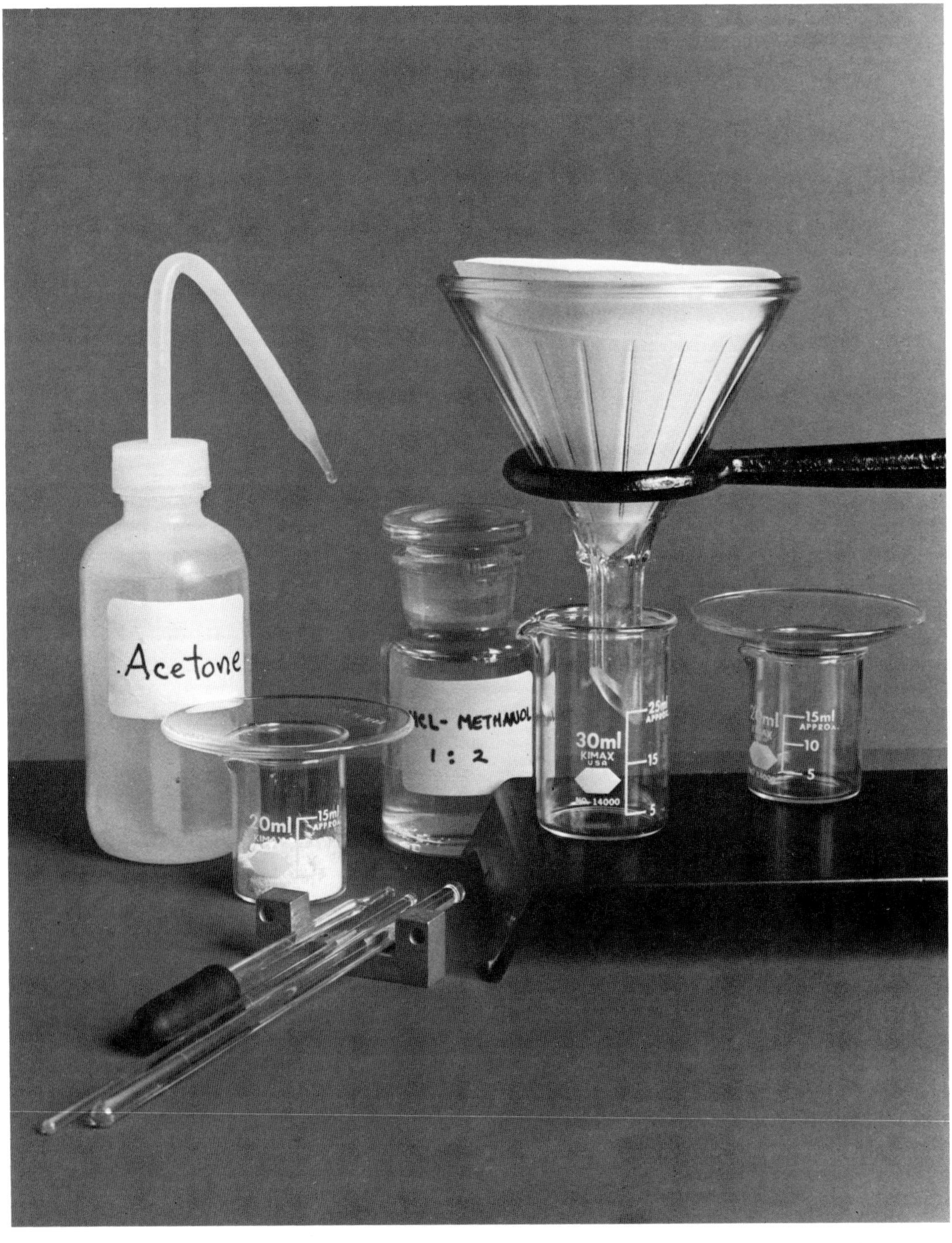

110. Equipment used for crystallization includes: one gram of cocaine base in a 20ml beaker covered with a watch-glass, acetone in a wash bottle, hydrochloric acid-methanol solution (1:2), filtration set-up with a 30ml beaker, a 20ml beaker with a watch-glass cover, two glass stirring rods, an eyedropper, a lab stand.

The Chemicals

The chemicals which are used to crystallize cocaine include:

1. The **solvent** in which the base is dissolved.
2. The **acid** which is used to lower the pH of the base solution.
3. The **solvent** which is used to dilute the acid.
4. The **solvent** which is used to wash the cocaine crystals after crystallization is complete.

The crystal growth will be affected by the *choice of solvents* and *acid* which are used. Also, the *purity* of the chemicals, the *temperature* at which they are used, and the *volumes* of each will greatly affect the outcome.

The Solvents

While the most commonly used solvent for cocaine crystallization is ether, it is extremely hazardous to use. Acetone, although highly flammable, is not as toxic as ether and does not form explosive peroxides. It works well for cocaine crystallization for the same reasons that it is effective as a wash. The base is extremely soluble in acetone, the hydrochloride is not. It evaporates completely, leaving no residue. Its major disadvantage is that, unlike ether, acetone will not have a visible white reaction to the addition of acid. This can make it difficult to determine the proper amount of acid to use and the point at which crystallization is complete.

The Acid

The name of the game is cocaine hydrochloride. It follows that the name of the acid is hydrochloric acid. When it comes as a liquid, hydrochloric acid can be 38% hydrogen chloride (HCl), no more. The remainder is water. Since the acid comprises only 1% of the total volume of liquid used to crystallize cocaine, this small

WARNING!

Some of the procedures documented, especially those involving volatile solvents or concentrated acids and alkalis may be extremely hazardous. The reader is cautioned not to perform any of these procedures. The procedures described should only be performed under laboratory conditions by professional chemists operating under the authority of the proper government regulatory agencies.

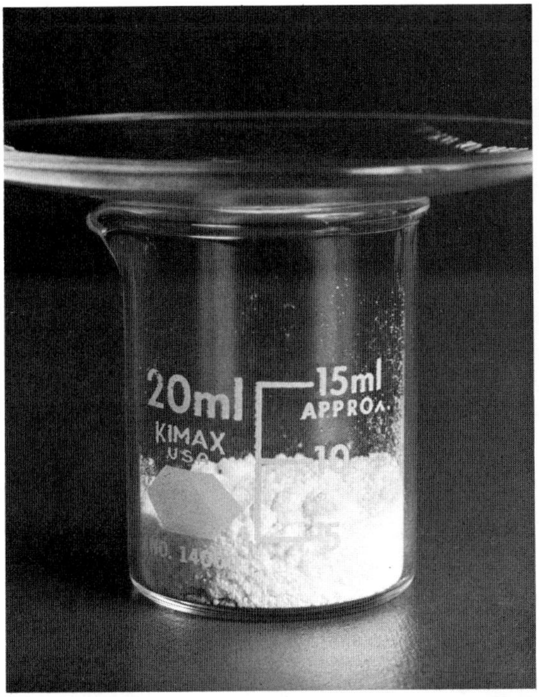

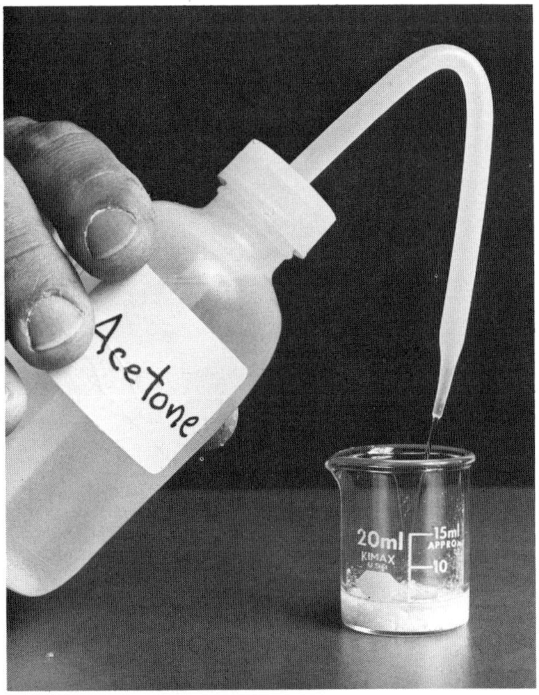

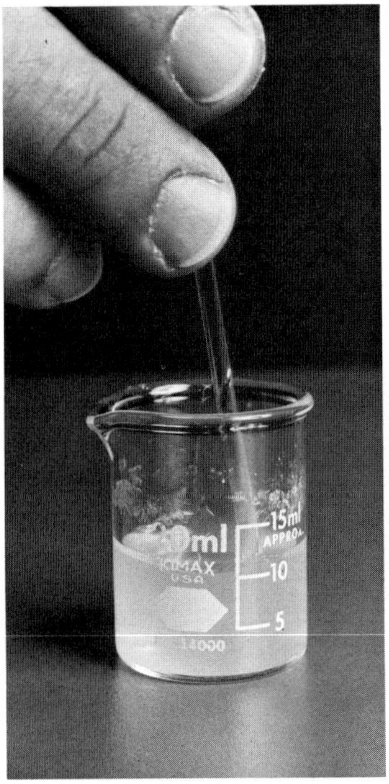

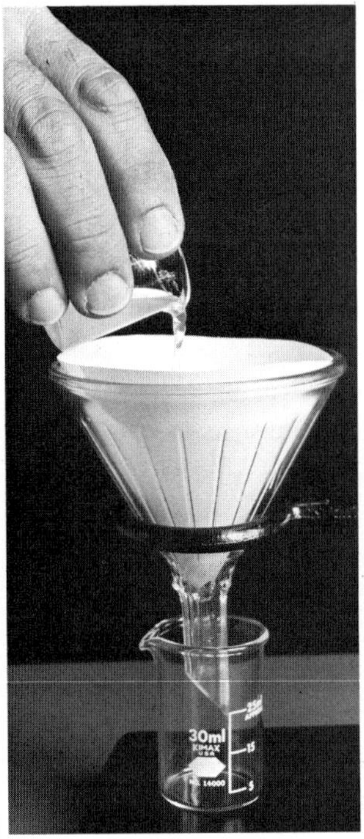

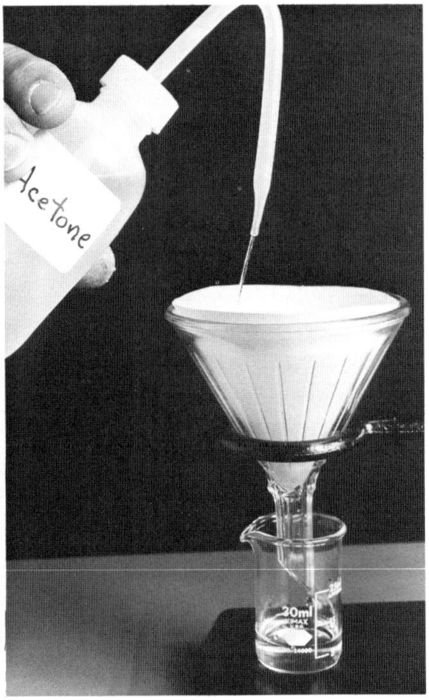

top:

111. One gram of cocaine base.
112. Ten milliliters of acetone is added to the gram of cocaine base.

bottom:

113. The acetone is stirred until the base is dissolved.
114. The liquid is filtered to obtain a clear solution.
115. The filter is rinsed to minimize any loss of the base and to increase the total volume of the solution to 15-20ml.

amount of water is not a problem. If, however, the acid were more dilute (with water) it would be a different story. For this reason, full-strength liquid hydrochloric acid is diluted with absolute methanol or acetone, or both.

The amount of hydrochloric acid which is needed to neutralize a given base will always vary with its alkaloid content and degree of alkalinity. In general, base which is made by the method described in the "Cocaine Base Test" (see p. 110) will require 0.25 milliliters of concentrated hydrochloric acid per gram of base. The amount is critical. If too much acid is used, the reaction will happen very fast. If too little, the reaction will be slow, and some base will remain in solution. In that case, more acid has to be added to complete the process. This will produce a secondary growth of crystals with characteristics different from those already formed. There is no all-encompassing formula. The exact amount of acid required is determined by trial and error using the above figures as a rough estimate (starting point).

Stirring

What may seem to be an insignificant detail is actually a prime factor in the rate of crystal growth. When the dilute acid solution (A) is added to the base/acetone solution (B), crystallization begins. The rate at which A is added and the time it takes for all of A to mix with all of B will significantly alter the rate of crystal growth. Ideally, solution B is swirled in a circular motion at a rate which will allow all of solution A to be added before B ceases to swirl. This allows the acid to be evenly combined with the base before much crystal growth has begun. If the acid is added after the swirling has stopped, it will sink to the bottom before mixing with the base and crystal growth will begin on the bottom. The result is usually trapped acid and uneven growth. If, on the other hand, swirling is continuous before, during, and after the addition of the acid, crystallization will be too rapid. While the resultant hydrochloride will be homogenous, the tiny crystals will lack the brilliance and clarity of more slowly grown crystals.

(Continued on page 169)

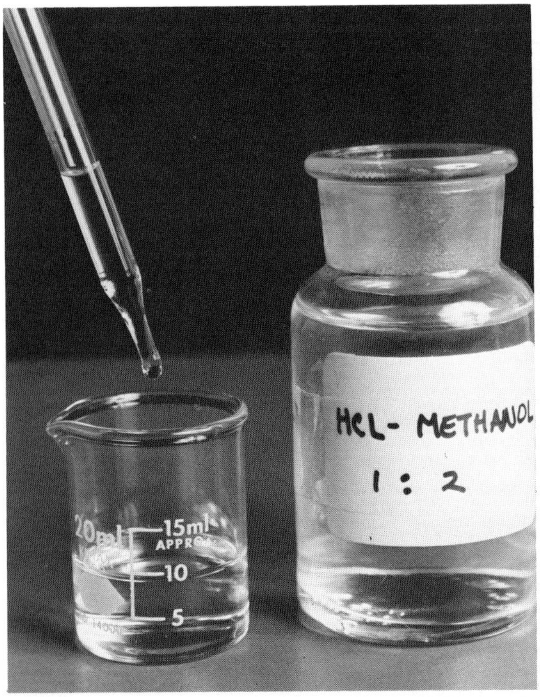

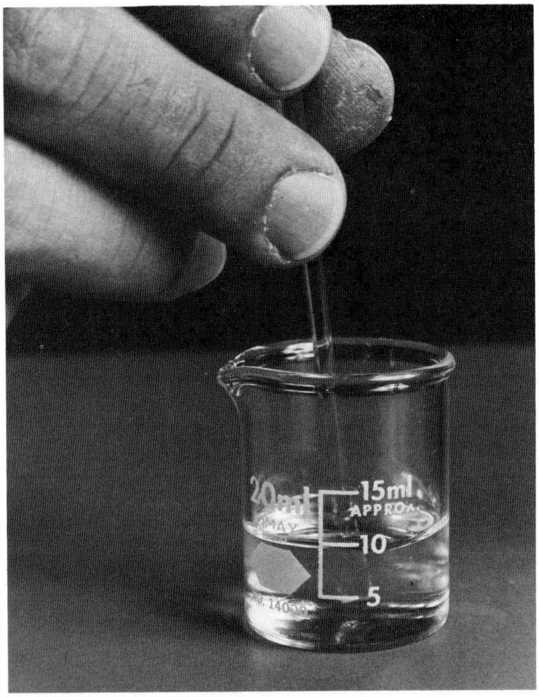

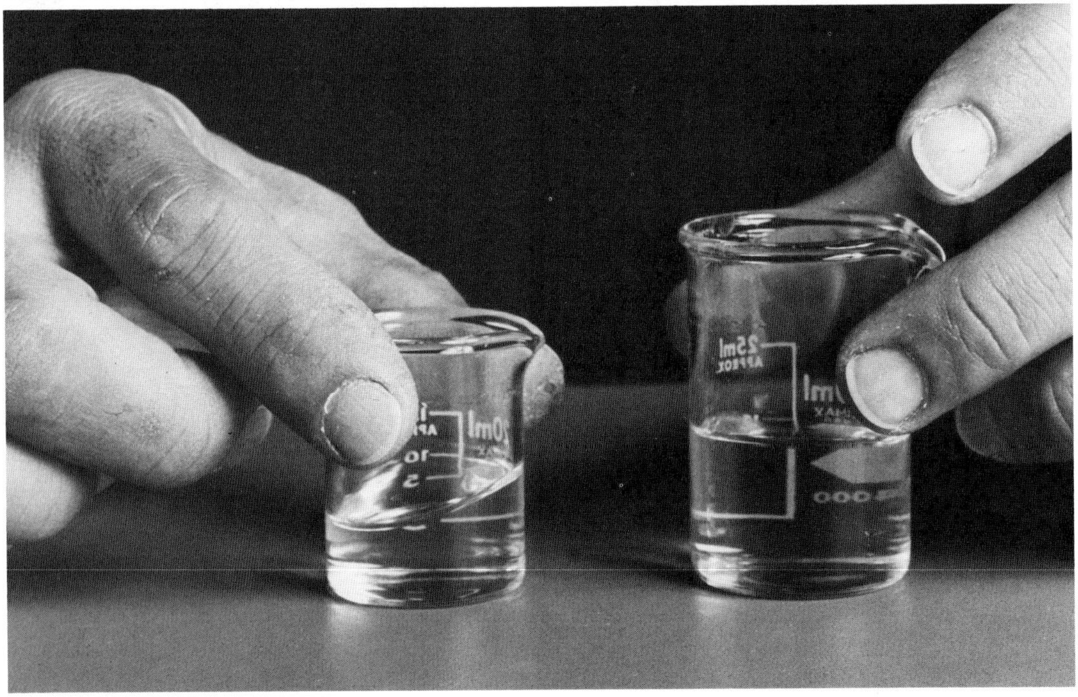

top:

116. In a separate beaker, about 25 drops (0.75ml) of the HCl-methanol solution is added to 10ml of acetone.

117. This acid-acetone solution is mixed well.

bottom:

118. The cocaine base solution and the acid-acetone solution are swirled simultaneously and in the same direction.

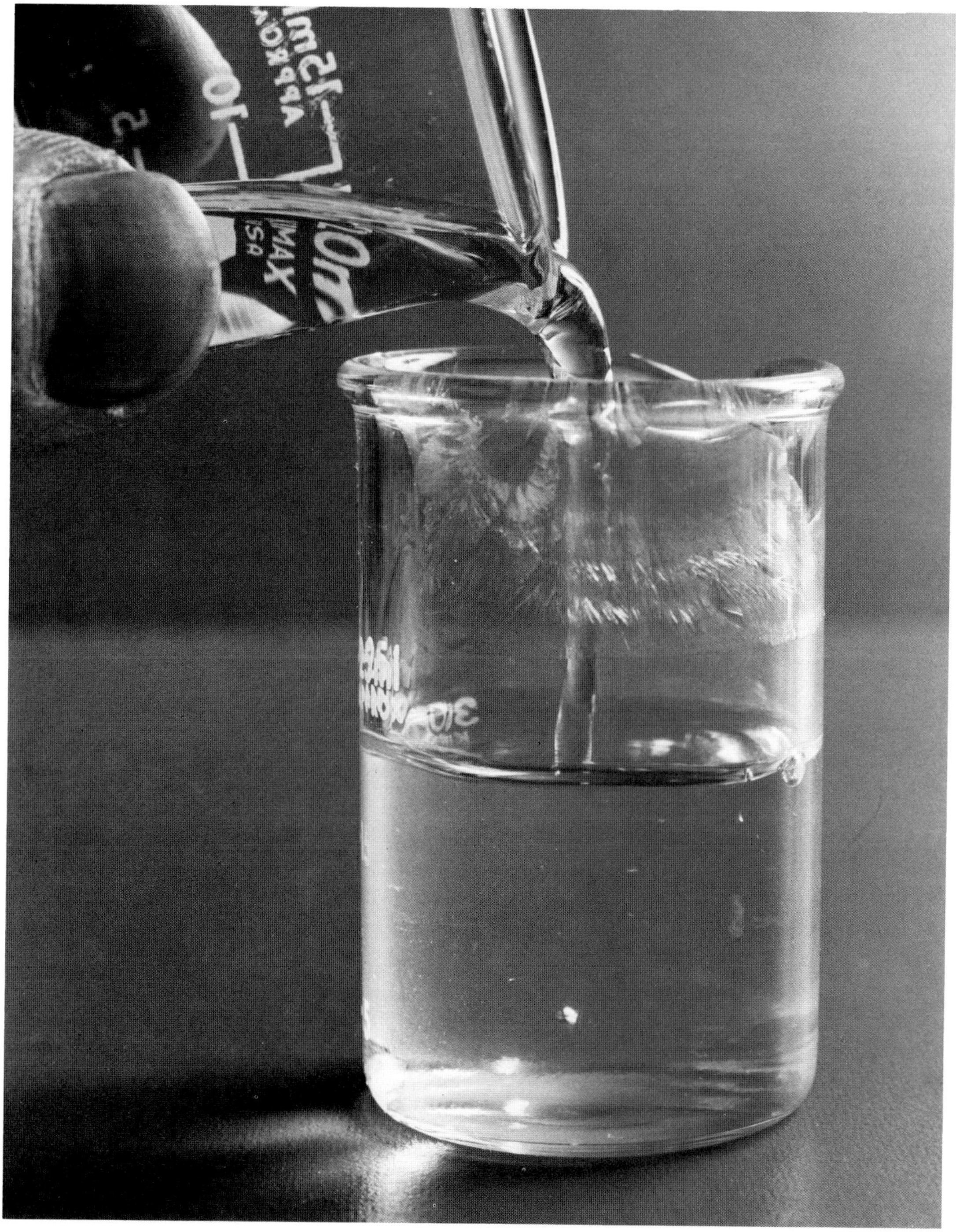

119. The acid-acetone solution is poured quickly into the cocaine base solution while both are still swirling.

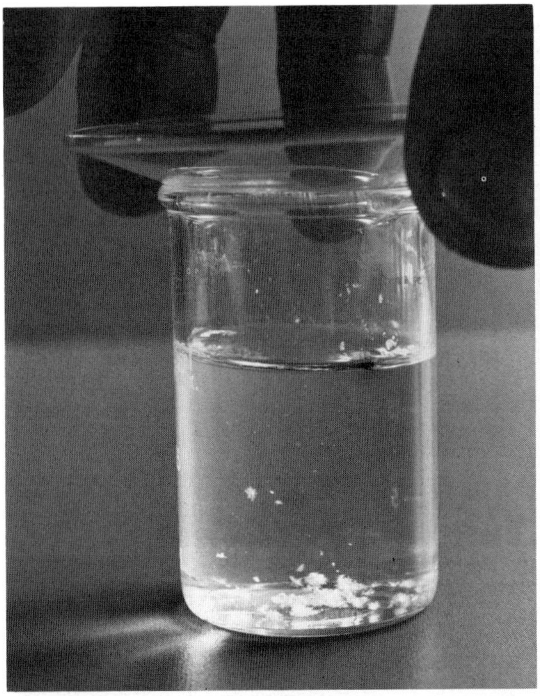

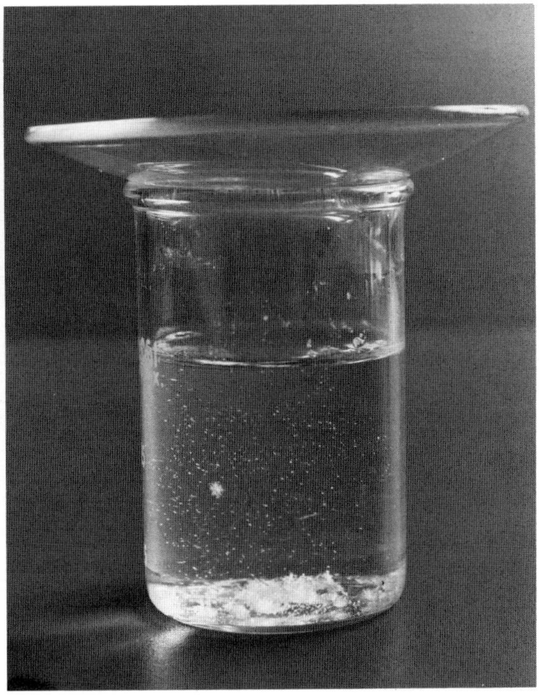

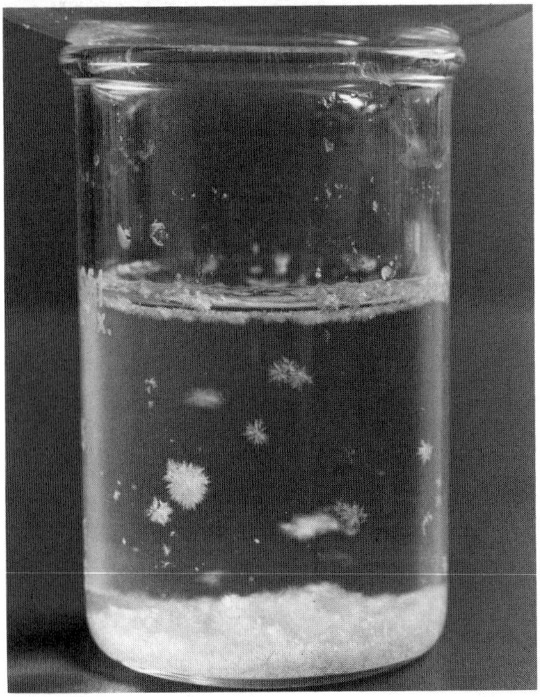

above:

120. By the time the solution is covered, cocaine hydrochloride crystals have begun to form.

121. Three minutes after mixing.

left:

122. Five minutes after mixing.

top row, opposite page:

123. Ten minutes after mixing (surface formation of crystals is falling to the bottom).

124. Thirty minutes after mixing: visible precipitation has stopped but the crystals continue to grow for several hours.

125. After two hours, crystals are stirred.

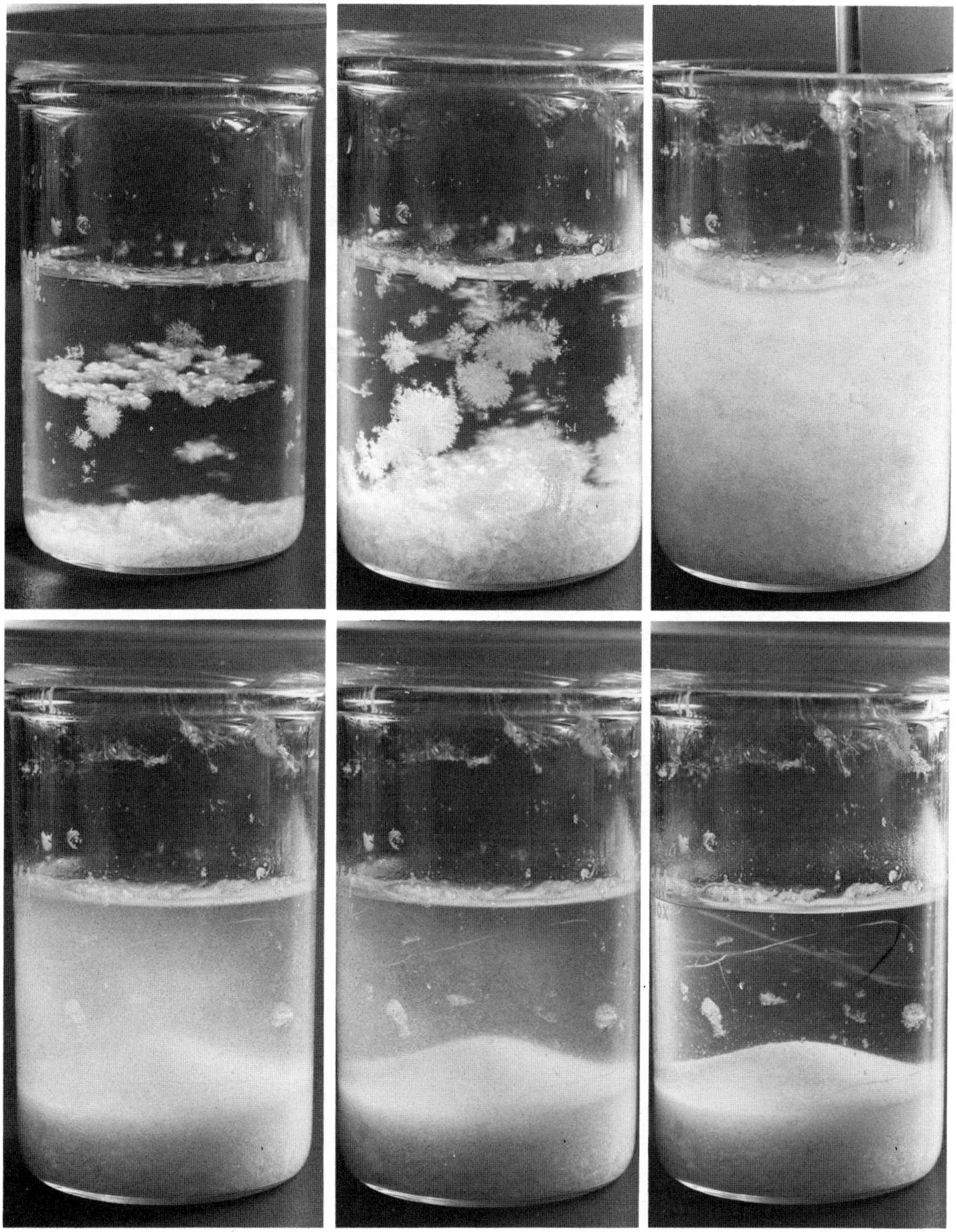

bottom row:

126. Crystals are allowed to settle.

127. The solution is still cloudy and new crystal growth is visible when the glass rod scratches the beaker. This indicates that crystallization was incomplete.

128. One hour after stirring, the solution has cleared and crystallization is finished.

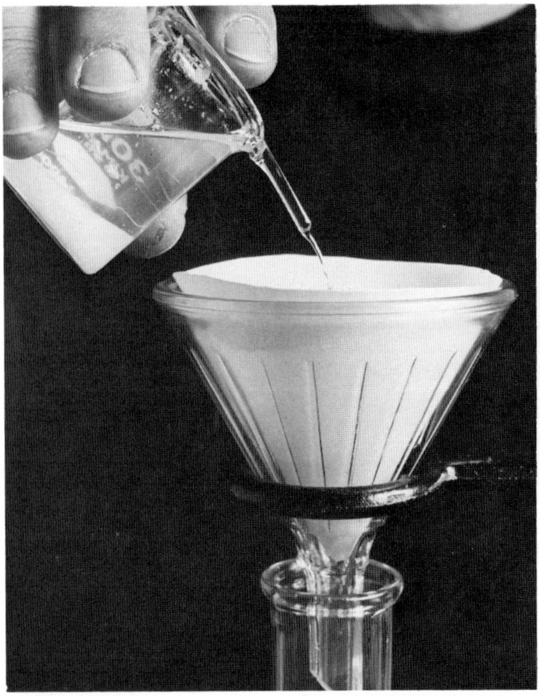

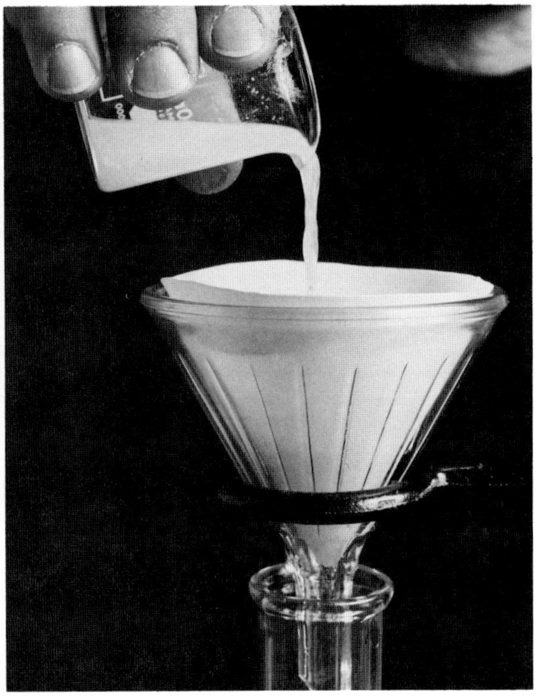

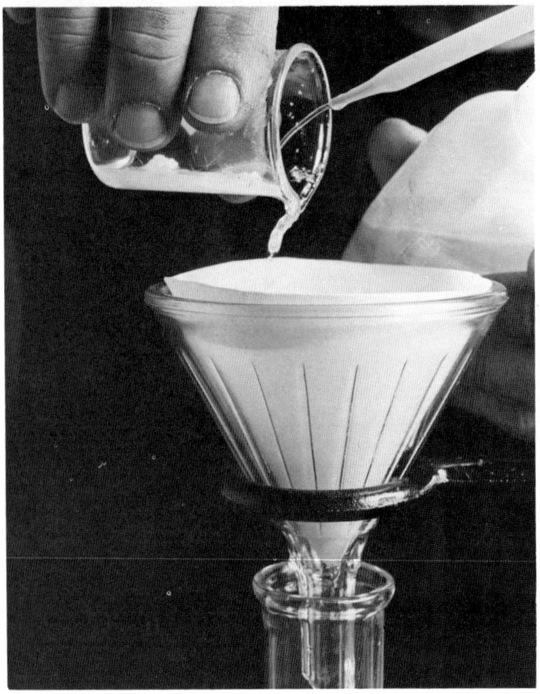

above:

129. The mother liquor is decanted from the crystals.

130. After two acetone washes by decantation, the final wash with the crystals is poured into the filter.

left:

131. The remaining crystals are rinsed into the filter with acetone.

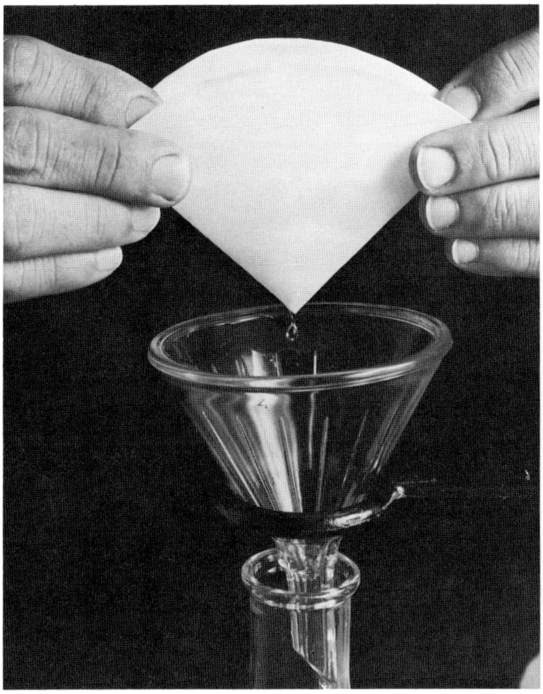

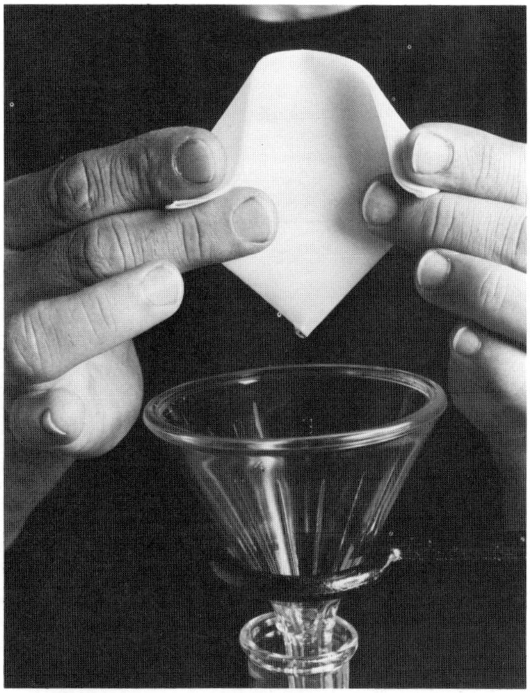

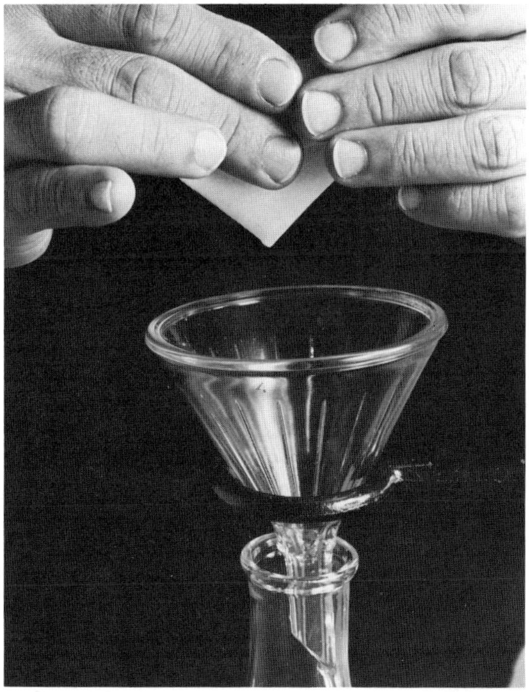

above:

132. After all the acetone has passed through, the filter paper is removed.

133. The sides are folded in.

right:

134. The top is folded down and the empanada is squeezed to press the cocaine hydrochloride crystals against one another while removing more solvent. It is then dried under a heat lamp.

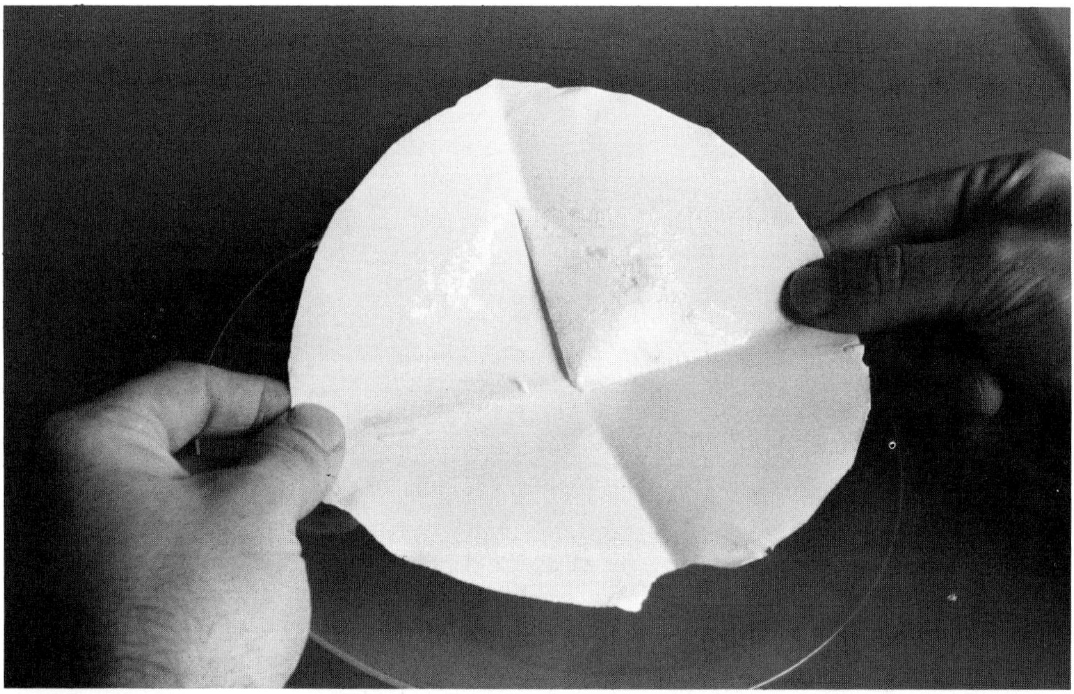

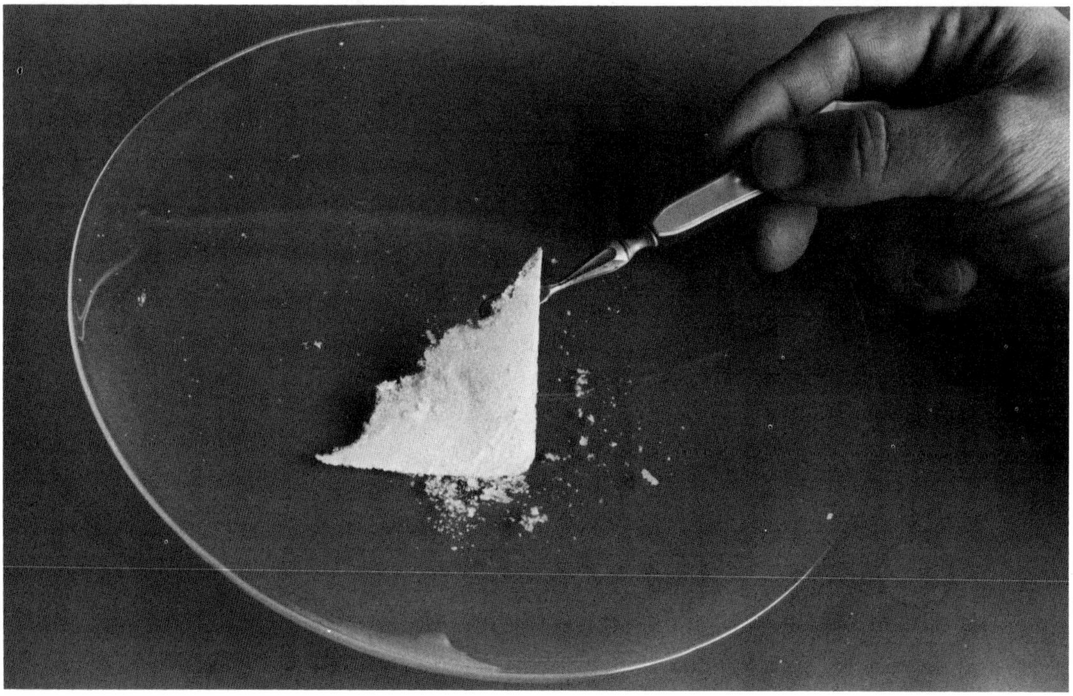

135. When the filter paper is dry to the touch, the empanada can be opened.
136. The flake is examined; the weight is one gram.

When is Crystallization Complete?

This is determined by trial and error. Generally, an acetone crystallization takes 4 hours. While there may be no more visible precipitation, this does not necessarily mean that crystallization is complete. This is characteristic of acetone crystallizations. The initial snowstorm (visible precipitation) may last only 15–30 minutes, but the crystals continue to grow in size and increase in weight for several hours thereafter. A determination must be made to see if crystallization is complete. This is accomplished by swirling the crystals and allowing them to settle. A completed crystallization will result in the cocaine settling to the bottom in a matter of minutes. The liquid above is clear. An incomplete crystallization leaves the liquid on top cloudy with falling crystals. The cloudiness will persist until crystallization is complete. If crystallization is incomplete and the side of the beaker is scratched with the stirring rod it will result in new growth where scratched.

Washing the Crystals

Once it has been determined that crystallization is complete, the mother liquor is separated from the crystals by decanting it into a separate container. Then, as in the acetone wash, fresh solvent is added to the crystals, swirled, and allowed to settle. This is decanted into the same container as the mother liquor. (This is because the first wash or decantation is rarely 100% effective in removing all of the mother liquor. The second decantation removes the remainder.) Again, fresh solvent is added, swirled, and the entire contents poured into the filter. The solvent is allowed to drip through before one last fresh portion of solvent is poured over the crystals. This completes the washing procedure.

Drying the Crystals (Making An Empanada)

In South America, crystal which is gravity filtered is dried "empanada style." This involves removing the filter cone, pressing it between the hands, and placing the damp empanada under a heat lamp to dry. This is not only the simplest way of drying the crystals with a minimum of contamination (remember that crystals are often dried outside in the sun), it is also the best way to make layered flakes.

Flakes are actually pressed crystals. If, as in an empanada, the crystals are pressed against one another and dried, the resultant piece of cocaine will have the texture of the filter paper on the outsides, and layers of pressed crystals (flakes) on the inside. When crystals are pressed or chopped, their brilliance increases. For this reason, the flake appears shinier than unpressed crystal. However, when the flake is chopped, it gets duller in appearance. In South America, where crystal is often dried in the sun, the filter paper acts as a protective shell, shielding the cocaine from dust and moisture. Sheets are often used instead of filter paper, and are hung on clotheslines to dry.

The timing of when to remove the filter cone from the funnel, and the force with which it is pressed, are the factors used to control the appearance of the empanada with varying types of crystal growth. When very small crystals are involved, layering is achieved by removing the filter cone just before all the solvent from the last wash has passed through the filter. Pressing is minimized to remove solvent only. The crystals are already small and if pressed too hard, the inside structure is usually that of unlayered rock. In the case of larger crystals, the empanada is squeezed firmly in order to flatten out the crystals. Often, the empanada is pressed between a piece of glass and filter paper. The extra filter paper acts as a firm ground on which to press the glass, and also as a blotter, absorbing excess solvent. Once pressed, the empanada is layed flat to dry.

It is critical that the filter paper be dry before the empanada is opened. Otherwise, some of the cocaine sticks to the filter paper and the consistency of the outside texture is imperfect. In South America, the empanada is allowed to stand at room temperature after the filter paper is dry. It is believed that continued heat after this point results in weight losses and overly dry cocaine. The fact is that dry is dry. When the weight ceases to change, the cocaine is dry.

THE END

APPENDICES

APPENDIX A

Discontinuing Cocaine Abuse

In any discussion regarding cocaine addiction, the problem is not the absence of facts; there are more than enough facts available. The problem lies in resolving the conflicts between the facts and relating them to the personal use of cocaine.

There seems to be no physical addiction. The physical effects of cocaine used in moderation are mild except when injected or used over extended periods of time. In *Licit and Illicit Drugs,* Edward M. Brecher states; "A cocaine user, even after prolonged use of large doses, does not, if deprived of his drug, suffer from a dramatic withdrawal syndrome. The physical effects of cocaine withdrawal are minor." This should not be interpreted to mean that no one becomes addicted to cocaine. It merely means that regular use of the drug does not create a physiological need for the drug.

Some people are content with occasional use of cocaine, while others acquire a habit. Of those that acquire the habit, some acquire it by inclination or preference and are able to discontinue use without severe discomfort. But what about those who feel compelled to use cocaine to the point of debilitation. If cocaine is not addicting, why are people drawn to its use? If the answer does not lie in the body, it must lie in the mind and in life.

The key to kicking any habit is personal desire. Until there is desire to quit smoking, drinking, cocaine use or television viewing, most attempts will end in failure. If you find you are afflicted with a cocaine habit, and you find it is hurting your life physically and spiritually, you must find and nurse the desire to stop the use of cocaine.

Sometimes it is hard to recognize such a habit. Mr. Brecher states that cocaine withdrawal "... is characterized by a profound psychological manifestation—depression—for which cocaine itself appears to the user to be the only remedy ..." In other words, 'coming down' from a cocaine high leaves you depressed, a depression you do not associate with the euphoric effects of cocaine. You feel the cocaine remedies this depression and fail to recognize that the depression is caused by the initial dose.

You should be aware of the effects of cocaine on mental processes. Louis Levin wrote a description of these effects in his 1924 book, *Phantastica:* "Will-power diminishes, and indecision, lack of a sense of duty, capricious temper, obstinacy, forgetfulness, diffuseness in writing and speech, physical and intellectual instability set in. Conscientiousness is replaced by negligence, truthful people become liars and the lover of society seeks solitude." Lewin's statement describes a composite effect. Not all people feel all these emotions; with some the effects are not pronounced; still others feel the effects quite intensely. If you have a cocaine habit, it is hard for you to view objectively the effect on your life. If you can't decide whether you are using too much cocaine; your indecision is a good indication that you are.

If you are an irrational or insecure individual, you may consider it impossible to discontinue cocaine use. You will have a tendency to feel you are incapable of quitting, so why try? Even if you understand the abuse of cocaine is detri-

---

This appendix originally appeared in the *Cocaine Consumer's Handbook* in 1976; it is worth repeating.

mental to your physical and mental health, you will feel compelled to snort. The best method of countering addiction is to remove yourself physically from cocaine and the environment that will give your cocaine habit reinforcement. Once this has been done, you must understand you may relapse if you are again exposed to cocaine use. Strive to improve your self-esteem and learn to feel secure about your own identity. Both steps are extremely hard and your success in this effort must depend greatly on the people closest to you. If you are rationally motivated, understanding your reasons for abusing cocaine may be sufficient for you to control or discontinue your habit.

There is also an addiction that springs from a life which is so boring, unfulfilling, unmotivated, miserable or poverty-stricken that you feel the only way you can tolerate life on a day-to-day basis is to alter your mental state with chemicals. This must be countered on both the personal and social level. If you are abusing cocaine because you find life boring or unmotivating, you have to realize the problem lies in your own perspective. The key lies in desire. If you desire a change in your drug habit, you must look for a way to change your life. You should combat boredom and lack of motivation by becoming involved in activities with people you admire, or which will give you personal satisfaction. The reinforcement you receive for your efforts will motivate you. The use of drugs in these instances will gradually be placed in perspective or discontinued. If your life is so miserable or poverty-stricken that you feel the need to use cocaine to enable you to cope with it, answers on a personal level are harder to find. If your condition of existence were improved, you would probably use cocaine sparingly as an occasional high or discontinue its use entirely. If it is in your power to improve your material position, you must have the desire.

When the power to improve your material position in life is not in your hands, there are other considerations. Governmental agencies, social agencies, and medical authorities approach the problem of drug abuse as basically caused by the properties of the drug. As long as this policy continues there will be widespread drug abuse. Only when meaningful attempts and coordinated efforts at improving the quality of life are made can there be progress made toward reducing or eradicating drug dependency. As long as these agencies are allowed to ignore that basic truth, they will continue to abrogate the responsibility placed in their hands by the people of this country.

In closing, reference can be made to a statement made by Richard T. Martin in his paper, "The Role of Coca in the History, Religion, and Medicine of South American Indians," published in *Economic Botany* #24, 1970: "The easiest way to resolve the conflicting reports on the effects of coca use is to recognize the fact that, like any other potent medicinal agent, coca is beneficial when used appropriately and is detrimental when used in excess."

APPENDIX B

Labs

This is a list of labs which do analysis of street drugs. When the use of illicit drugs expanded in the '60s the problem of adulteration and misrepresentation became common and about a hundred labs started operating to provide accurate information as to the contents of street drugs. Restrictive legislation and official pressure has reduced the number to 9; 7 do it on an anonymous basis, but for 2 the sample must be delivered in person. Fees range from free to $15.00 a sample and the time necessary after they get the sample varies from one day to 2 weeks. Only qualitative (what's in it, not how much of each) results are given since it is now illegal to provide any quantitative information to the general public.

The time needed to get results from these labs means that they would probably not be much help to testing quality before purchase. When a dealer has stock to sell it's usually available for only a short time so it would all be sold by the time the analysis is done. The main use could be to check the quality of something a consumer is about to use, or has used. The accuracy of these labs has been questioned from time to time; one way of checking this might be to send the same sample to several of the labs and see if they agree.

CALIFORNIA

- **Los Angeles County Dept. of Drug Abuse**
  Director: Sallie Montgomery
  849 South Broadway, 11th Floor
  Los Angeles, CA 90014
  213-974-7680

The Program: This is a very large program. They have referral services for treatment and various drug-related problems. The referral telephone number is 213-974-7659. They have a lab and it is an anonymous service.

The Procedure:
(this service is for L.A. County residents only)
- This is a free service
- Must be street drugs (no unknowns or prescribed drugs)
- Must be identified as what you think it is
- Must be well packaged and padded
- Must give sample a random identification number
- Must be sent certified mail to:
  Medical Receiving
  1410 Biggy Street
  Box J6
  Los Angeles, CA 90033

Obtaining Results: It takes different amounts of time for processing but usually 2-3 days. Call 213-974-7680 and give the random identification number, the certified mail number receipt, and what you think the drug is.

- **Pharm Chem Foundation**
  Director and Publisher of newsletter:
  David Ogden
  3925 Bohannon Drive
  Menlo Park, CA 94025
  415-328-6200 (new number)

The Program: They have been in business for 10 years.

The Procedure:
- Fee is $15 (money order)

- Send 25 milligrams (1/8 tsp.) wrapped in aluminum foil
- Assign sample a code number (5 random numbers followed by 1 letter of the alphabet)
- Mail the sample in a padded envelope (mark HAND CANCEL)

Obtaining Results: It takes 2 days for processing, then call their phone number listed above and give the code number; results will be given over the phone.

Test results summarized in PharmChem newsletter, published 10 times yearly.

FLORIDA

- **UpFront Incorporated**
  Co-ordinator: Carolyn J. Ciancutti
  P.O. Box 330589
  Coconut Grove, FL 33133
  305-446-3585

The Program: This is a drug information center with a watts line for information in Florida which is 1-800-432-8255. It is private, non-profit and funded by the State through the Drug Prevention Program. Their lab, which is the only one in Florida for street drug analysis, is:

S.P. Lab
1800 N.W. 10th Avenue
Miami, FL 33130

The Procedure:
- $10 fee (analysis is anonymous)
- Send 1 tablet, or 1 joint or 3 match heads (size) of powder
- List what you think the sample is and any of the undesirable effects
- Assign it a 5-digit code number
- Wrap the sample in aluminum foil
- Write HAND CANCEL on package to protect the parcel from being crushed

Obtaining Results: It takes 5-7 working days for analysis. Then call 305-446-3585 and give the code number. They will give results over the phone.

ILLINOIS

- **Street Drug Analysis Service**
  Director: Kenneth R. Lohr
  1301 Broadway
  Quincy, IL 62301
  217-223-7040
  217-223-7041

The Program: This service has existed for 24 years. The director is a pharmacist who feels that it is important to get bad drugs off the streets.

The Procedure:
- This is a free service
- Strictly anonymous
- Send (1 dose) wrapped in foil (cocaine would be 1/8 to 1/4 tsp.)
- Assign it a code number, either numerical or letter

Obtaining Results: It takes 24 hours upon receiving the sample to process it. With the mail it can take 7-10 working days to receive results. Call in for results and give the assigned code number, or you can send a stamped self-addressed envelope for return of results.

MARYLAND

- **Community Counseling & Resource Center**
  Director: Beverly Grady
  517 Virginia Avenue
  Towson, MD 21204
  301-628-6120

The Program: This program has been in existence for 10 years. It is an outpatient facility with a laboratory. It is non-profit and funded by the United Way and Drug Abuse Council.

The Procedure:
- This is a free service
- The sample *must* be brought in person to the center to be analyzed; a code number is assigned at that time

Obtaining Results: Results can be obtained by phone or mail for $.50.

MINNESOTA

- **Metro Drug Awareness** (for high school students with cocaine problems)

Director: Ron Friye
250 South 4th St.
Minneapolis, MN 55415
612-348-8027

The Program: This is a referral center which focuses on prevention, education and consulting. They do have a laboratory, and they are funded by the State.

The Procedure:

- This is a free service
- Send the sample to:
  Metro Drug Awareness
  Street Drug Lab
  Room 505 (at the above address)
- Done anonymously, assign it a 4-digit code
- Wrap the sample in plastic or aluminum foil
- Information to be put on the sample is:
  Cost of sample
  State, city or area the sample came from
  Symptoms or side effects of the sample
  Whether samples sent by a counselor, user, teacher
- Write on the front and back of the package: HAND CANCEL

Obtaining Results: Analysis takes 1 to 2 weeks. Phone in for results 612-348-8027 and give code number.

OHIO

- **Drug Analysis Unit**
  Director: Jim Young
  Free Medical Clinic
  12201 Euclid Avenue
  Cleveland, OH 44106
  216-721-4010

The Program: The drug analysis unit began 1965/66 and the free medical services began in 1970. It is funded privately and all the procedures are provided free of charge.

The Procedure:

- This is a free service
- All aspects are anonymous
- Locals can walk in and set up service anonymously
- The sample is to be wrapped in aluminum foil or plastic, assigned a code number and mailed to the above address

Obtaining Results: Results are given over the phone, call 216-721-4010 and give the identifying number.

- **United Health Service**
  Director: Russell Falck
  184 Salem Avenue, Suite 228
  Dayton, OH 45406
  513-225-3003

The Program: This is a referral service for treatment, etc. which has been in existence for 10 years. It is mostly an educational, consulting and training center funded by the State. They do have a lab service but it is regional (in 3 counties).

The Procedure:

- This is a free service
- Drop off service (no mail)
- The sample is given a code number

Obtaining Results: They only do qualitative analysis which takes 72 hours. Phone in for results.

WASHINGTON

- **Street Drug Analysis Laboratory**
  Director: Dr. Galpin
  College of Pharmacy
  Washington State University
  Pullman, WA 99164
  509-335-5676

The Procedure:

- This is a free service
- Send tightly closed plastic bag with contents
- Put down what the contents are supposed to be
- Include city or area of origin
- Include street price
- Assign the sample a code number taken from serial number on a dollar bill

Obtaining Results: Analysis takes 9 days to 2 weeks. If you want results returned, send a self-addressed stamped envelope, or call in to 509-335-4773 and give serial number of package.

APPENDIX C

Health Centers

Problems associated with cocaine abuse vary with the particular situation. Individuals with an overdose problem are advised to go directly to a hospital emergency room. For less acute problems of abuse there are thousands of public and private treatment and counseling centers in the U.S. Individual states publish a resource directory of such centers and it may be obtained by writing to the state's department of health and welfare. The telephone directory lists *crisis intervention agencies* in the front of the book and many communities also have a "hot line" which can locate such centers. Many options are available, so shopping around is probably a good idea. Fees for public organizations are often on a sliding scale—from free up, depending on income. Group therapy can be as low as $20.00 a week. Private care is usually more expensive but sometimes a sliding scale of fees also operates. In-hospital care can range from $350 to $4000 a week.

A survey of about 100 centers across the U.S. indicated that the pattern of abuse was remarkably similar everywhere in the country; Abuse of cocaine alone is hardly ever seen, usually a number of drugs, alcohol, barbiturates, heroin and others are involved. Most public centers encounter alcohol and heroin abuse problems—a very low percentage is concerned with mainly cocaine—although when questioned what drugs the individual uses, cocaine is frequently among those mentioned.

The consensus of these centers is that regular cocaine use is mainly a characteristic of the middle class and the well-to-do, particularly in the entertainment industry. It is an expensive habit but also one which allows the individual to function at a job (unlike alcohol and heroin). Abuse is almost always connected to some personal problem and crisis—drug consumption increases, this causes additional psychological and physical problems which the drug seems to alleviate, so consumption increases even more. The high financial cost of the habit adds to this psychological pressure. This cycle is characteristic of what the counselors call an addictive personality. Since the abuser of cocaine is usually well-to-do, any professional assistance they seek is likely to be from a private physician or institution; getting an estimate of the extent of the abuse problem is difficult.

Prominent individuals, mostly entertainers, who have gone public about their cocaine abuse, produce instant media attention and undeniable proof that cocaine abuse can produce horrible results. Alcohol abuse produces physical and psychological damage on a massive scale but public revelation of an alcohol problem produces only passing media interest. In effect, the media, by such reactions, are creating a glamour around what is mainly a personal tragedy. It is very unlikely that anyone of prominence will go public about their moderate use of cocaine. But the question remains, how are the 20 million Americans who consume cocaine using it, and how big is the problem of cocaine abuse?

ARIZONA

- **Tucson 24-Hour Crisis Line**
  Help-on-Call
  602-323-9379 for counseling and referrals

- **Center for Counseling**
  Director: Perk Clark
  40 E. 14th Street, #8
  Tucson, AZ 85701
  602-792-3130

  Fee: Sliding Scale

  Service: Out-patient counseling for poly-drug problems, referrals.

  Comments: Staff counselors have M.S.W.'s and M.A.'s, has been in existence for 4 years.

CALIFORNIA

- **Project Eden**
  Telephone counseling line for drug overdose and information (24-hour service)
  415-538-3818

- **Change**
  Director: Rudi Glover
  2880 Sacramento St.
  Berkeley, CA 94702
  415-845-7320

  Service: Out-patient counseling and drug education and treatment; referrals; staffed by clinical psychologists.

- **Project Concern**
  Director: Joan Alsop
  3220 Sacramento St.
  Berkeley, CA 94702
  415-655-2575

  Service: Referral service; crisis counseling for drug-related problems.

- **Do It Now Foundation**
  Director: Sandy Coburn
  6136 Carlos Avenue
  Hollywood, CA 90028
  213-463-6851 (24-hour crisis line)
  213-462-7131

  Service: Out-patient counseling and treatment center for poly-drug problems, drug-free counseling; referrals.

  Comments: Considered among the best in the L.A. area. Staffed by psychologists and out-patient counselors. They will refer people to M.D.'s or medical facilities.

- **Women's Substance Abuse and Resource Center**
  Director: Leslie Bragg
  543 North Fairfax, Room 306
  Los Angeles, CA 90036
  213-653-2005

  Service: Out-patient counseling and referrals for poly-drug problems.

- **Los Angeles County Dept. of Drug Abuse**
  Director: Sallie Montgomery
  849 South Broadway, 11th Floor
  Los Angeles, CA 90014
  213-974-7659

  Service: This is a very comprehensive resource. They can refer one to various treatment facilities and referral services in the L.A. area for drug related problems; they also have a lab to test street drugs.

- **Narcotics Education League**
  Director: Juan Covarrubias
  3315 East 14th Street
  Oakland, CA 94601
  415-536-4760

  Service: Out-patient counseling program which uses a therapeutic approach of support-groups of ex-addicts; also offers employment help and training; education.

- **Oakland Community Counseling**
  Director: Dr. Janet Leckner, Ph.D.
  341 MacArthur Blvd.
  Oakland, CA 94610
  415-839-1010

  Service: Referral; poly-drug counseling (drug-free counseling).

- **Cabrillo Medical Center**
  Director: John Milner
  CARP Program
  3475 Kenyon Street
  Point Loma, CA 92106
  714-222-0411, ext. 370

  Fee: Take medical insurance

  Service: Out-patient counseling for poly-drug problems.

- **Crisis Hot Line for the San Diego Area**
  714-352-7873

  Service: They act as a referral service; they refer the following:
  - **Pathway Central** at 714-297-3927
  - **House of Metamorphosis** at 714-234-4628
  - **Maac Regional Counseling Center** at 714-429-7670

- **Haight/Ashbury Clinic**
  Director: Dr. Darryl Inaba
  529 Clayton Street
  San Francisco, CA 94117
  415-621-2014

  Fee: Free with donations

  Service: Out-patient counseling and de-tox program; acupuncture treatment and medication are used for getting people off drugs; psychological counseling program as well.

- **Delancy Street Foundation**
  2563 Divisadero Street
  San Francisco, CA 94115
  415-563-5326

  Service: This is a residential treatment program and they will not accept anyone who is not already drug-free; psychological approach used to find out what causes patients to be addictive personalities.

- **Palmer Drug Abuse Program**
  5605 Woodman Avenue, Suite 209
  Van Nuys, CA 91401
  213-989-0902

  Area Served: Los Angeles, Sherman Oaks, and Beverly Hills

  Fee: None

  Service: Out-patient counseling staffed by ex-addicts that have been through a 12 step process.

COLORADO

- **Comotis Crisis Center**
  Director: Richard Barnhill
  9840 East 17th Avenue
  Aurora, CO 80040
  303-343-9890 (24-hour crisis line for the Denver area)

  Service: Telephone crisis counseling and referrals; walk-in counseling service for drug-abuse problems.

- **Denver University Open Clinic**
  303-753-3245 (24-hour hot line during school session)

  Service: Provides information on legal issues and telephone counseling about drug-related problems.

- **The Cocaine Clinic**
  Director: Dr. Anker, Clinical Psychologist
  1827 Gaylord Street
  Denver, CO 80206
  303-388-5894 (24-hour answering service)

  Service: Out-patient clinic; treats addiction and provides counseling; research being conducted about cocaine and the results of the addiction.

  Comments: Staffed by psychiatrist, psychologist and some M.A.'s. They also have a branch of the clinic in Aspen, Colorado.

- **Substance Treatment Center**
  Director: Dick Robbins
  2475 West 25th Avenue
  Denver, CO 80211
  303-455-2251

  Fee: $25 per week

  Service: Out-patient counseling center; treats poly-drug abusers; has counseling and referral service.

  Comments: Staffed by nurse, psychologist, and mental health counselors.

- **Palmer Drug Abuse Treatment Program**
  12900 West Alameda Parkway
  Lakewood, CO 80228
  303-989-8015

  Fee: None

  Area Served: Denver, Wheatridge, Evergreen, Northglen, Longmont and Boulder

  Service: Out-patient counseling staffed by ex-addicts who have been through a 12-step program for at least one year.

CONNECTICUT

- **Branford Counseling Center**
  33 Laurel Street
  Branford, CT 06405
  203-481-4248

  Service: Provides out-patient counseling for drug-related (and other) problems and referrals; from 9 A.M. to 5 P.M., Monday through Friday.

- **Information Line for Hartford**
  203-521-7150 for referrals and counseling (telephone)

- **Institute of Living**
  400 Washington Street
  Hartford, CT 06106
  203-278-7950

  Fee: Sliding scale based on income.

  Service: Out-patient and residential facilities for poly-drug abuser, treatment and counseling, individual psychotherapy.

  Comments: Non-profit private institute in existence for 25 years.

- **The High Intervention Program**
  New Haven, CT
  203-789-7389

  Service: Counseling and treatment for poly-drug abusers.

- **Connecticut Mental Health Center**
  34 Park Street
  New Haven, CT 06511
  203-789-7282

  Service: Out-patient poly-drug treatment and counseling, general counseling and referrals.

FLORIDA

- **Switchboard of Miami**
  305-358-HELP (24-hour crisis line)

  Service: Provides telephone counseling and referrals for drug problems and other crises.

- **Pact**
  30 Southeast 8th Street
  Miami, FL 33131
  305-358-1640

  Service: Out-patient counseling and therapy for poly-drug problems, family counseling, individual therapy.

- **Palmer Drug Abuse Program**
  2635 Cleveland Avenue
  St. Meyers, FL 33901
  813-337-2898

  Fee: None

  Service: Out-patient counseling staffed by recovered drug-abusers and alcoholics who have participated in a 12-step program for at least one year.

GEORGIA

- **Midtown Intake Center**
  Director: Mr. Carrol Benson
  22 - 8th Street
  Northeast Atlanta, GA 30309
  404-894-4561

  Service: Out-patient counseling for poly-drug problems, detoxification program, referrals.

HAWAII

- **Honolulu Crisis Line**
  808-521-4555

ILLINOIS

- **Gateway House Foundation** (administration office)
  Director: John Sabora
  Executive Director: Michael Darcy
  624 South Michigan
  Chicago, IL 60605
  312-663-1130

  Area Served: Illinois

  Fee: Donations

  Service: Referral and poly-drug treatment program for adults, three residential treatment programs, one out-reach program. Counseling and treatment.

- **Alternatives, Inc.**
  Director: Bruce Kuehl
  1126 West Granville

Chicago, IL 60626
312-973-5400

Area Served: Chicago

Service: Out-patient care and counseling for ages 12-14 years, drug-free treatment.

INDIANA

- **Mid-Town Drug Free Program**
  Director: Lee Bjerki
  155 East Market St., Suite 810
  Indianapolis, IN 46204
  317-630-6991

  Area Served: Regional

  Fee: Sliding scale based on income.

  Service: Poly-drug treatment center, individual and group counseling.

  Comments: Open Monday through Friday 8 A.M. to 5 P.M.

IOWA

- **Des Moines Crisis Linė**
  515-262-9551

- **Des Moines Drug Information Line**
  515-280-1111

  Service: Provide information about street drugs and referrals for counseling and poly-drug treatment.

LOUISIANA

- **Louisiana Mental Health Association Crisis Hot Line**
  504-524-COPE for counseling and referrals

- **New Orleans 24-Hour Crisis Hot Line**
  504-523-2673 for referrals

- **New Orleans Substance Abuse Center**
  Administrator: Duane Belgard
  3934 Canal Street
  New Orleans, LA 70119
  504-568-5531

  Fee: Sliding scale based on income.

  Service: Out-patient clinic, counseling and treatment for poly-drug abusers; alcohol, smoking, and weight problems. Offer individual therapy, family therapy, group and couple counseling.

  Comments: One of the biggest and most comprehensive programs in the state of Louisiana, staffed by social workers, nurse, doctor, and two consultant psychiatrists.

MARYLAND

- **State of Maryland Drug Abuse Administration**
  Herbert O'Conner Building
  Maryland Dept. of Health and Mental Hygiene
  201 W. Preston Street, 4th Floor
  Baltimore, MD 21201
  301-383-3312

  Service: Information about treatment programs and organizations which offer services for drug abusers; referrals.

- **Community Counseling and Resource Center**
  Director: Beverly Grady
  517 Virginia Avenue
  Towson, MD 21204
  301-823-4357

  Service: Out-patient counseling center which offers referrals, general counseling for drug problems, and lab.

MASSACHUSETTS

- **Project Place**
  32 Rutland Street
  Boston, MA 02138
  617-262-3740 (business line)
  617-267-9150 (hot line)

  Fee: Sliding scale based on income.

  Service: General counseling and referral, crisis hot line, crisis intervention.

  Comments: They referred to two clinics, which they considered outstanding for drug problems in Boston.

  - **Boston Addiction Services**
    617-436-6000

  - **Boston University Drug Clinic**
    617-247-6415

- **Bridge Over Troubled Water**
  23 Beacon Street
  Boston, MA 02108
  617-227-7114 (24-hour crisis line)

  Fee: Sliding scale based on income.

  Service: Drug-free counseling and out-patient center for poly-drug problems.

- **Survival Drug Treatment Center**
  1354 Hancock Street
  Quincy, MA 02169
  617-471-7100 (24-hour crisis hot line)
  617-471-8400

  Service: Offers out-patient counseling and treatment for adolescents, and crisis line.

MICHIGAN

- **Drug Abuse and Suicide Prevention Crisis Line**
  Detroit, MI
  313-875-5444 (24-hour)

- **Project Headlines**
  Administrative Director: William Sumner
  15085 East 7 Miles
  Detroit, MI 48205
  313-526-5000 (24-hour hot line)
  313-526-6000

  Area Served: Detroit and the county

  Service: Seven programs—crisis, out-patient counseling, after-care, residential treatment and detoxification.

  Comments: This state/county program has existed for 10 years. They reported that Detroit has a growing cocaine problem and that a wide variety of help is available throughout the city for anyone who is serious about solving their problems.

MINNESOTA

- **Metro Drug Awareness**
  Director: Ron Friye
  250 South 4th Street
  Minneapolis, MN 55415
  612-348-8027

  Service: Referral center which focuses on prevention, education, consulting, training, short-term crisis counseling, and intervention for drug problems; they also have a lab.

  Comments: They referred to these other centers for help in drug related problems:

- **Minnesota Growth Exchange**
  Director: Bruce Henney
  501 West St. Germain, Suite 319
  St. Cloud, MN 56301
  612-253-0930

- **Minnesota Institute on Black Chemical Abuse**
  Director: Peter Bell
  612-871-7878

- **Chrysalis Center for Women**
  Director: Kathy Zimorsiak
  612-871-0118

MISSOURI

- **Acid Rescue**
  Executive Director: Heidi Israel
  11745 Olive Street Road, Suite 205
  Creve Coeur, MO 63141
  and
  1408 North King Highway
  St. Louis, MO 63113
  314-569-2161 (also a 24-hour hot line)

  Fee: Sliding scale based on income

  Service: Referral, drug-free out-patient counseling and treatment for poly-drug problems.

  Comments: In existence since 1968, staffed by six counselors and one nurse.

- **Kansas City Hot-Line for Drug Abuse**
  816-836-8572

- **Nasco**
  Director: Dr. William M. Harvey
  2305 St. Louis Avenue
  St. Louis, MO 63106
  314-436-2832 (24-hour crisis line)
  314-241-4310

  Fee: Sliding scale based on income

  Service: Out-patient treatment center for poly-drug problems, this facility offers an 18-month to 2-year rehabilitation program.

NEVADA

- **Fitzsimmons House**
Executive Director: Dick Steinberg
900 East Karen, Suite A112
Las Vegas, NV 89109
702-737-7601

Area Served: Western United States

Fee: Sliding scale based on income

Service: Poly-drug counseling, residential treatment program, referrals, and day-care center.

- **Theraputic Associates**
Paul Casey: Sole Proprietor
3101 Maryland Parkway
Las Vegas, NV 89109
702-735-2057

Area Served: Nevada

Fee: About $35.00 for an individual counseling session.

Service: This is a private office with a staff of five counselors and a psychologist for consultation. They provide poly-drug counseling.

Comments: Method used is reality therapy from the Institute of Reality Therapy in Los Angeles, CA.

- **Western Counseling Associates**
Director: Roger Hosker
900 East Karen, Suite C215
Las Vegas, NV 89109
702-369-5700

Area Served: Western United States

Fee: Sliding scale based on income

Service: This is the out-patient clinic of Fitzsimmons House. Poly-drug counseling and therapy staffed by licensed professionals and psychologists.

NEW JERSEY

- **Englewood Drug Abuse Program**
75 Englewood Ave.
Englewood, NJ 07631
201-569-4442

Service: Counseling and referrals.

- **DARE**
(Drug Addiction Rehabilitation Enterprise)
Out-Reach Center
87 N. Day St., Orange, NJ 07050
201-678-7065
Residence
209-211 Littleton Ave., Newark, NJ 07103
Residence
19 High St., Orange, NJ 07050
201-642-7411
24-hour hot line
201-673-0636

Area Served: All of New Jersey

Fee: None

Service: Drug-free counseling and referral; medical care, encounter groups, counseling for personal problems. Three-stage complete rehabilitation program for those who need and want it.

- **Damon House Out-Reach**
363 Broadway
Patterson, NJ 07501
201-742-3733

Fee: None

Service: Out-patient counseling and group and individual care for persons of any age.

- **Damon House**
Director: Ted Dequercio
369 Market Street
Patterson, NJ 07501
201-279-5563
and
105 Joyce Kilmer Ave.
New Brunswick, NJ 08901
201-828-6002

Fee: None

Service: Residential treatment program (drug-free) for persons of any age.

Comments: Staff of counselors, ex-addicts and psychologists.

- **Corner House**
273 Witherspoon Street
Princeton, NJ 08540
609-924-8018

Area Served: Mercer County

Fee: Sliding scale based on ability to pay

Service: Non-residential, drug-free counseling and referral; day-care facilities.

- **Fair Oaks Hospital**
  Director: Dr. Mark Gold
  19 Prospect St.
  Summit, NJ 07901
  201-277-2300

  Area Served: Unrestricted

  Fee: One of the more expensive private facilities in the U.S.A. Most insurance companies' hospitalization covers the costs.

  Service: Residential program and out-patient care utilizing new non-opiate treatments for addicts.

  Comments: This treatment was developed by Fair Oaks physician-researchers at Yale and Fair Oaks. Specially trained staff work closely with family and as a referral source to prevent relapse.

- **Riverview House**
  5700 Boulevard East
  West New York, NJ 07093
  201-861-9600

  Area Served: West New York

  Fee: None

  Eligibility: Not physically addicted to a drug

  Service: Non-residential, drug-free group and individual therapy, various workshops, and referrals.

  Procedure: Interview includes evaluation; if rejected, individual is referred to other facility.

- **Junction**
  1040 Asbury Ave.
  Ocean City, NJ 08226
  609-398-1700
  and
  2507 New Jersey Avenue
  Wildwood, NJ 08260
  609-729-1663

  Area Served: Cape May County

  Fee: None

  Service: Out-patient direct counseling, psychological counseling, drug-free rehabilitation, inmate counseling.

- **Private Practitioners in the NJ Area**

  Ralph Barracano, M.S.
  9 Zachary Lane, Apt. 4
  Groveville, NJ 08620
  215-637-2324 (answering service)
  609-585-3685 (appointments)

  Area Served: Unrestricted

  Fee: By the office visit

  Service: Licensed psychologist, treats poly-drug problems, counseling.

  R.C. Skadegaard, M.S.
  110 Valley Road
  Watchung, NJ 07060
  201-561-6368

  Area Served: Unrestricted

  Fee: By appointment

  Service: Therapist that treats poly-drug problems, counter-culture therapist.

NEW MEXICO

- **Drug Counseling Program**
  Director: Rick Miera
  1330 San Pedro N.E.
  Albuquerque, NM 87110
  505-266-8784

  Fee: Sliding scale based on income

  Service: Poly-drug treatment program, both out-patient and residential, individual and group therapy, referrals.

  Comments: Staffed by therapists with master's degrees working under the supervision of a psychiatrist. They have four offices located around the city.

- **La Saliba**
  Director: Manuel Chavey
  P.O. Box 2673
  North Highway 85
  Las Vegas, NM 87701
  505-425-7572

Service: Poly-drug counseling and treatment, personality testing, and training for jobs.

Comments: This program is very much like the Delancy Street Foundation in theory and practice. They do not believe in using ex-addicts as counselors and provide a professional staff.

NEW YORK

- **Daytop Village**
  54 W. 40th Street
  New York, NY 10018
  212-564-1834 (information line)
  212-564-1838 (hot line)

  Area Served: New York City

  Service: Treat all drug abuse problems, staff consists of professionals and ex-addicts; out-patient counseling and therapy; they also have five residential treatment facilities in upstate New York. (Have seven different locations in New York City for out-patient counseling.)

NORTH CAROLINA

- **Raleigh North Carolina Crisis Line**
  919-782-3060

- **Drug Action**
  919-832-8686

OHIO

- **United Health Service**
  Director: Russell Falck
  184 Salem Avenue, Suite 228
  Dayton, OH 45406
  513-225-3003

  Area Served: Regional, three counties

  Service: Referral service for poly-drug treatment, educational, consulting and training center.

OKLAHOMA

- **Palmer Drug Program**
  210 S.E. 9th Street
  P.O. Box 295
  Bartlesville, OK 74003
  918-336-0921

  Fee: None

  Service: Out-patient counseling program, staffed by recovered drug-abusers/alcoholics who have participated in a 12-step program of training for at least one year.

OREGON

- **Lane County Mental Health Division**
  Director: Jim Lakehomer
  Drug Program
  1901 Garden Avenue
  Eugene, OR 97403
  503-687-4000 (8 A.M. to 12 P.M.)

  Service: Drug-free counseling program for poly-drug problems and a methadone maintenance, referrals.

  Comments: They have licensed professionals and psychologists.

- **Comprehensive Options for Drug Abuse**
  Director: Patrick Vanzo
  Supervisor: Terry Jenkins
  Drug Treatment Services
  7305 N.E. Glisan
  Portland, OR 97213
  503-257-0533

  Fee: Sliding scale based on income.

  Service: Poly-drug out-patient center, counseling and referrals.

PENNSYLVANIA

- **Center for Addictive Drugs**
  Director: Dr. Connell
  Paoli Memorial Hospital
  #5 Industrial Blvd.
  Paoli, PA 19301
  215-648-1130

  Service: Out-patient treatment providing counseling and therapy for poly-drug abusers.

- **The Institute of the Pennsylvania Hospital**
  Director: Dr. Edgar Nase, Psychiatrist
  The Strecher Program
  111 North 49th Street
  Philadelphia. PA 19139
  215-829-2711
  215-829-2701

Fee: Approximately $25 for group therapy per week, and about the same for an individual private session.

Service: Comprehensive treatment program for alcohol and poly-drug problems, group therapy and individual psychotherapy, with family involvement.

Comments: Staffed by psychiatrists, M.D.'s, and psychologists.

- **Clear Brook Lodge**
  Director: Frank Babowicz
  R.D. #2, Box 146A
  Shickshinny, PA 18655
  717-864-3116

  Area Served: They take people from all over the United States.

  Fee: Most people use their medical insurance to pay.

  Service: In-patient facility (in the beautiful mountains of upstate Pennsylvania) treats assorted drug and alcohol problems. The program is a 42-day treatment for drugs, and the facility will provide the patient with an after-care follow-up program arranged at the patient's home. This is a drug-free treatment counseling program.

  Comments: They have the capacity to treat 70 people at the lodge and have a private plane which can arrange to pick up people all over the country.

TENNESSEE

- **Sumner Co. Guidance**
  Director: C. Gordon
  528 E. Main Street
  Gallatin, TN 37066
  615-259-3754

  Fee: Sliding scale based on income

  Service: Out-patient center; it provides counseling for early addiction relating to poly-drug problems; handles crisis calls.

  Comments: Open 8 A.M. to 5 P.M.

- **Drug Abuse & Referral Line**
  Nashville, TN
  615-254-6547

- **Crisis Intervention**
  250 Venture Circle
  Nashville, TN 37228
  615-244-7444

  Service: Trained volunteers answer the 24-hour line and provide referral and telephone counseling.

- **National Drug Treatment**
  700 Craig Head Avenue
  Nashville, TN 37205
  615-327-3521

  Service: Out-patient poly-drug counseling facility; referrals.

  Comments: They have been treating a large number of cocaine problems. In existence for about 9 years, they are open 12 hours a day.

- **Mid-Cum Council A & D**
  250 Venture Circle
  Nashville, TN 37228
  615-254-6547

  Fee: Free

  Service: Consultations and referrals; education, prevention, and counseling.

TEXAS

- **Freedom Connection**
  Director: Clarence Leopold
  2340 Rosewood
  Austin, TX 78702
  512-472-6261

  Area Served: Austin area

  Fee: Intake fee, and weekly fee based on income

  Service: Comprehensive poly-drug treatment program, out-patient care and counseling, referrals, and methadone program.

  Comments: In existence for 9 years; have a resident psychologist.

- **Help Is Possible**
  Director: Bill Watkins
  3603 Ross Avenue
  Dallas, TX 75204
  214-827-2870

Fee: None

Service: Drug-free counseling for all drug-abuse problems. Similiar in theory and practice to Synanon using peer pressure.

Comments: In existence since 1973, and is a federally funded program.

- **Houston Crisis Line**
713-228-1505

- **Texas Research Institute of Mental Sciences (TRIMS)**
Director: Dr. Tim Sharma, M.D.
1700 Holcolmb
Houston, TX 77030
713-797-9752

Area Served: All of Texas

Fee: Sliding scale based on income

Service: Comprehensive poly-drug treatment program; out-patient and residential, chemical-free treatment.

- **Palmer Drug Abuse Program**

313 North Center Street
Arlington, TX 76011
817-277-0111

Area Served: Fort Worth, and Arlington

510 W. 35th Street
Austin, TX 78752
512-458-6361

Area Served: Austin, includes Georgetown, Waco and San Marcos

600 Belmead Drive
Corpus Christi, TX 78412
512-993-0495

3966 McKinney
Dallas, TX 75204
214-526-8110

Area Served: Dallas, includes Plano, Carrollton, Longview, Dangerfield, and Tyler

6221 Main Street
Houston, TX 77030
713-524-1868

Area Served: Houston, Stafford, Conroe, Huntsville, Spring, Victoria, Lake Jackson, LaMarque, Pasadena, Port Arthur, and Beaumont.

P.O. Box 10396
Midland, TX 79702
915-685-3645

Area Served: Midland, Odessa and San Angelo

301 W. Russell Place
San Antonio, TX 78212
512-733-6171

Area Served: San Antonio, and New Braunfels

Palmer's National Information Number
713-977-6436

Administrative Office for the West
Palmer Drug Abuse
6400 West Park, Suite 250
Houston, TX 77057
713-977-8334

Fee: None

Service: Out-Patient counseling program; staffed by recovered drug-abusers/alcoholics who have participated in a 12-step program for at least one year.

UTAH

- **Drug Referral Center**
Director: Michael Dercaria
146 East 6th South
Salt Lake City, UT 84111
801-355-7413

Fee: Sliding Scale

Service: Referral service, information. Out-patient service which gives out information about drugs and drug programs; provides psychological evaluations.

- **Community Crisis Center**
Director: Bob Terrheno
327 East 6th South
Salt Lake City, UT 84111
801-355-2846

Fee: Donations

Service: Drug-free counseling center treating poly-drug abusers, and other problems. Referrals.

Comments: Private, non-profit out-patient center. In existence for 12 years. Staffed by four counselors with M.A.'s.

VIRGINIA

- **Crisis Center Referral Service**
  Richmond, VA
  804-780-8004

- **Project Jump Street**
  Director: Wesley Stuart
  15 West Cary Street
  Richmond, VA 23220
  804-644-4636

  Fee: About $7.50 a week

  Service: Out-patient counseling and poly-drug treatment; residential treatment program; methadone maintenance program; and drug-free counseling.

  Comments: Staffed by four counselors, three nurses, one doctor, and a psychiatrist.

WASHINGTON

- **Seattle Crisis Intervention Hot Line**
  206-687-4115

- **Substance Abuse Recovery Program**
  Director: Jane Middelton
  1600 East Olive Street
  Seattle, WA 98122
  206-281-4323

  Service: Out-patient poly-drug treatment program that operates five days a week.

WISCONSIN

- **Crisis Intervention Line**
  Madison, WI
  608-251-2345 (24-hours)

- **PICADA (Prevention and Intervention of Alcohol and Other Drug Abuse)**
  Director: Julie Pfeifer
  17 North Webster Street
  Madison, WI 53703
  608-251-4558

  Area Served: Dane County

  Fee: Free

  Service: Information and referrals, short term counseling for poly-drug abusers, counseling and education.

  Comments: Private non-profit drug abuse center.

- **Dane Co. Mental Health Center**
  Director: Robert Mohelnitzky
  31 South Henry
  Madison, WI 53705
  608-251-2341

  Area Served: Dane County

  Service: Poly-drug counseling and therapy, referral.

- **Crisis Intervention Line**
  Milwaukee, WI
  414-257-7222 (24-hours)

- **Underground Switchboard**
  Financed by the Milwaukee Council on Drug Abuse
  414-271-3123 (24-hours)

- **Rehabilitation Hospital**
  Referred by Underground Switchboard
  414-271-7822

- **The Counseling Center**
  Director: Ted Seaver
  1428 North Farwell Avenue
  Milwaukee, WI 53202
  414-271-4610

  Fee: Free

  Service: Eight session counseling program, referrals for poly-drug problems, also general counseling.

Glossary

A

absolute (alcohol) - 100% (alcohol), anhydrous, having no trace of water in it

acetone - a flammable organic solvent often used as a degreasing cleaner—it mixes with water in all proportions

adulterant - a substance added to a sample to decrease the concentration of the original material

agua de coca - water infusion of coca leaves, drunk as a tea in South America

alkaloid - a nitrogen-containing organic compound which reacts like a base, examples are caffeine and cocaine

ammonium hydroxide - the basic compound which results when ammonia gas reacts with water—it is the active ingredient in household ammonia cleaner

amphetamine - a synthetic central nervous system stimulant—the word "speed" and amphetamine are almost synonymous

B

base smoking - the heating of cocaine base to vaporize it and inhaling the vapors—usually done in a glass pipe

baseable - the property of a compound which will make it soluble in an organic solvent like petroleum ether when the pH is made basic

benzocaine - a synthetic local anesthetic with a melting point of 88-92°C

benzoic acid - an organic acid which is one of the building blocks of the cocaine molecule

benzoylecgonine - a combination of benzoic acid and ecgonine—each is a building block of the cocaine molecule

Bolivian style cocaine hydrochloride - also known as "Bolivian rock"—a dense crystal-like form of illicit cocaine hydrochloride—the origin is not necessarily Bolivia

butacaine - a synthetic local anesthetic, the sulfate has a melting point of 138.5-139.5°C

C

caffeine - an alkaloid which is a stimulant and found in coffee, tea and numerous other plants (mp 238°C)

capillary tube - when referring to melting point tests, it is the thin-walled tiny glass tube which is filled with powdered sample and observed while heating

Cheyne-Stokes respiration - a pattern whereby breathing builds deeper and deeper to a point, then becomes progressively shallower, with a period of no breathing between cycles

cinnamylcocaine - an alkaloid related to cocaine where cinnamic acid replaces benzoic acid in the molecule

Clorox test - a method used to test cocaine for adulterants which uses a glass of liquid laundry bleach (5.25% sodium hypochlorite)

coca - a shrub originating in the Andes from which the alkaloid cocaine is derived

cocaine - the alkaloid obtained from coca leaves which has activity both as a local anesthetic and a stimulant of the central nervous system

cocaine base - the form the cocaine molecule has in a basic solution having no electrical charge; it is soluble in organic solvents

cocaine hydrochloride (pharmaceutical) - a salt form of pure cocaine which has an electrical charge and is soluble in water

cocamine (truxillines) - a group of alkaloids related to cocaine in structure but not having the pharmacological activity of cocaine

crystal - for cocaine, refers to cocaine hydrochloride

crystal lab - an illicit lab, usually in South America, which converts cocaine base into cocaine hydrochloride

cut - slang for adulterant

D

DEA - the acronym for Drug Enforcement Administration

duff - term used to describe the fine powder which passes through a screen when a sample is gently shaken

E

ecgonine - the central molecular building block of the major coca alkaloids, from the Greek for son or descendant

empanada - the form the crystals of cocaine hydrochloride take after drying inside the flattened filter paper, the appearance being similar to a South American meat pie

Erythroxylum coca - one of the species of coca

Erythroxylum novogranatense - one of the species of coca

Erythroxylum truxillense - one of the varieties of coca

ether (diethyl) - the solvent traditionally used to make cocaine hydrochloride; this ether is extremely flammable and forms explosive peroxides on exposure to air

F

flake cocaine - a form of cocaine hydrochloride that appears to be made of many paper thin layers of pearly crystals, sometimes "Peruvian flake"; it is more properly Peruvian style flake since it refers to the form rather than the country of origin

foil burn test - a test for cocaine hydrochloride adulterants where a small sample is heated from below on a sheet of aluminum foil

forensic (labs) - refers to an argument used in court, as a lab it usually means a police lab

freebase - the slang term for the alkaline form of the cocaine molecule (*not* the salt form) which is used for smoking

G

gas chromatograph(y) - a usually analytic technique which separates a mixture of compounds from each other in a stream of moving gas which passes through a specially designed tube

H

Huanaco - a region in South America where a species of coca is thought to originate

hygrines - a group of coca alkaloids which are oily bases

I

inositol - a type of sugar-alcohol (mp 225-227°C) which is frequently used to adulterate cocaine hydrochloride

Ipadu (or Amazonian) coca - one of the species of coca

L

lactose - a sugar also known as milk-sugar (mp 201-202°C) which is sometimes used to adulterate cocaine hydrochloride

lidocaine - a local anesthetic (mp 68-69°C) frequently used to adulterate cocaine hydrochloride or sold as cocaine hydrochloride itself

M

mannitol - a sugar-alcohol (mp 166-168°C) which is currently the most commonly seen adulterant of cocaine hydrochloride

mass spectrometer (high resolution) - an analytical tool which fragments and separates molecules into various building blocks which can frequently provide enough information to reconstruct what the original molecule looked like

melting point - the temperature or range of temperature at which a solid turns to a liquid

melting point test - the determination of the melting point or range of a sample to estimate its degree of purity; impurities lower the melting point and widen the range of the melting point

methanol - methyl alcohol,also known as wood alcohol, a poisonous flammable solvent

methyl benzoate - a compound with a strong wintergreen aroma; it is produced when cocaine is heated with absolute methanol in a basic solution

mother-of-pearl cocaine - cocaine hydrochloride crystals in flake form which have the appearance of mother-of-pearl

N

non-baseable - the chemical characteristic of an adulterant which leaves it in the water phase when the cocaine base is filtered or extracted with organic solvent

P

pasta - cocaine sulfate (with other alkaloid sulfates), a water soluble salt produced in an early stage of refining illicit cocaine

pasta lab - the lab, usually in South America, where coca leaves are brought to be turned into pasta

Peruvian style cocaine hydrochloride - a flake form of cocaine hydrochloride crystals which in the past was thought to originate in Peru; now it refers to the form of crystal; the alkaloid can come from anywhere

petroleum ether - not a true ether but a fraction of petroleum distillation, similar to gasoline in chemistry

pH - a scale used to measure acidity, pH 1 is extremely acidic, pH 14 extremely basic, and pH 7 is neutral

phenylpropanolamine - a compound (mp 101-101.5°C) used in antihistamines and non-prescription diet pills, similar to amphetamines in chemistry and sometimes used to adulterate cocaine

potassium permanganate - a chemical which is frequently used to oxidize and break down organic compounds; in refining cocaine it can be used to eliminate non-cocaine alkaloids

Potpourri - a mythical country or region where many samples of illicit cocaine really originate; most cocaine now results from leaves gathered from diverse regions

procaine - a local and spinal anesthetic (mp 61°C) sometimes used to adulterate cocaine

Q

quinine - an alkaloid from cinchona bark usually used to treat malaria; the sulfate is sometimes used to adulterate cocaine, and is dangerous to the user

R

rock cocaine - a form of cocaine hydrochloride which is dense, unlayered, and similar in appearance to rock salt

S

snorting - taking a drug by inhalation through the nose

spectrophotometer - an optical instrument which reads how much light of a particular wavelength a sample absorbs

T

tetracaine - a local anesthetic (mp of hydrochloride, 147-150°C) sometimes used to adulterate cocaine

Thiele-Dennis tube - a special glass tube used in in determination of melting points; it allows slow, even elevation of temperature

thin-layer chromatography - usually analytical method for separating a mixture into its pure compounds; it uses a thin, solid film on a plate and a special solvent which slowly moves across the plate and moves the different compounds different distances

tropacocaine - one of the alkaloids in coca which is related to cocaine

truxillic acid - one of the building blocks of alkaloids related to cocaine; they take the place of benzoic acid in cocaine

W

wash - the process of mixing a solid and solvent which will not dissolve the solid and separating the liquid and solid by decantation or filtration; impurities soluble in the liquid are removed in the process

Bibliography

Andrews, G., and Solomon, D., eds. 1975. *The coca leaf and cocaine papers.* New York: Harcourt Brace Jovanovich.

Antonil, 1978. *Mama coca.* London: Hassle Free Press.

Ashley, R. 1975. *Cocaine, its history, uses and effects.* New York: Warner Books.

Brecher, E.M., and Consumer Reports, eds. 1972. *Licit and illicit drugs.* Boston: Little Brown and Co.

Byck, R., ed. 1974. *Cocaine papers–Sigmund Freud.* New York: Meridian.

Chasin, D. 1974. *The gourmet cokebook, a complete guide to cocaine.* Washington, D.C.: White Mountain Press.

Crowley, A. 1973. *Cocaine.* San Francisco: Level Press.

Gottlieb, A. 1976. *The pleasures of cocaine.* Manhattan Beach, CA: 20th Century Alchemist.

Grinspoon, L., and Bakalar, J.B. 1976. *Cocaine, a drug and its social evolution.* New York: Basic Books.

Helmer, J. 1975. *Drugs and minority oppression.* New York: Seabury Press.

Martin, R.T. 1970. The role of coca in the history, religion and medicine of South American Indians. *Economic Botany* 24(4): 422-38.

Meyer, N. 1975. *The seven percent solution.* New York: Ballantine Books.

Mortimer, W.G. 1974. *History of coca.* Berkeley, CA: And/Or Press.

Mule, S.J., ed. 1976. *Cocaine: chemical, biological, clinical, social and treatment aspects.* Cleveland: CRC Press.

Phillips, J.L., and Wynne, R.D. 1980. *Cocaine, the mystique and the reality.* New York: Avon.

Pitigrilli, 1975. *Cocaine.* Berkeley, CA: And/Or Press.

Plowman, T. 1979a. Botanical perspectives on coca. *Journal of Psychedelic Drugs* II (1-2): 103-17.

______. 1979b. The identity of Amazonian and Trujillo coca. *Botanical Museum Leaflets of Harvard University* 27(1-2):45-61.

Sabbag, R. 1976. *Snow blind.* New York: Avon.

Szasz, T. 1975. *Ceremonial chemistry.* Garden City, N.Y.: Anchor Press.

Woodley, R. 1975. *Dealer: portrait of a cocaine merchant.* New York: Warner Books.

Younger, E.J., ed. 1975. *Stimulants. Part II of drug and user identification series.* State of California Department of Justice Division of Law Enforcement Advanced Training Center.

Index

A

Abstinence, from cocaine use, 16, 48
Acetone, 89-90, 137, 138, 150-2, 153, 155, 159, 160, 161, 162-4, 169; safety, 12
Acetone wash, 147-55, 166, 169; equipment, 148; procedure, 149, 150-2
Acid, in crystallization, 159, 161, 162-3
Adulterants and adulteration, 19, 43, 44, 45, 46, 70-5, 79, 80, 83, 146-7; melting points, 107; solubilities, 89-90. *See also* Cutting, of cocaine
Aesthetics, 52, 79, 153, 155, 156, 157, 161
Aging process, in acetone wash, 155
Agua de coca, 24
Alcohol poisoning, 50
Alcohol use, 57; with cocaine, 50, 54; as solvent, 155
Alkaloids, in coca, 24, 25, 30, 31, 32-9, 40; in cocaine, 79, 104
Amazonian coca (var. of *E. coca*). *See Ipadu coca*
Ammonium hydroxide, 52, 110, 111, 112, 114, 116, 122, 155
Amphetamine, as adulterant, 72, 85, 107; detection in tests, 89, 97, 142-3, 144-5
Amphetamine, as stimulant, 57
Anesthetics, as adulterants, 71, 74, 100. *See also* specific anesthetics
Aphrodisiac, coca as, 24, 25. *See also* Sex and cocaine

B

Barbiturates, 57
Base labs, 35-6, 41, 42, 45
Benzene, 89-90, 155
Benzocaine, 74, 89, 100, 107
Benzoic acid, 34, 37, 38
Benzoylecgonine, 32, 34, 38, 39, 89, 107, 134
Bernhardt, Sarah, 26
Bindle, 44, 78, 79
Black market. *See* Cocaine market
Bleach. *See* Clorox test
Bolivia, 23, 25, 30, 35, 41
"Bolivian rock" cocaine, 83, 85, 94, 133, 142-3, 144-5
"Book standard" (of cocaine), 83, 93, 142, 144-5
Borax, 15, 72
Brazil, 25, 29, 30
Butacaine, 74, 89, 107
Buyers (of coca), 41, 45

C

Caffeine, as adulterant, 14, 72, 84, 100, 107; detection in tests, 89, 97, 99, 144-5
Caffeine, as stimulant, 57, 60
Carbon disulfide, 89-90
Cheyne-Stokes breathing, 57
Chloroform, 89-90
Chuspa (coca pouch), 131
Cinnamic acid, 38
Cinnamylococaine (alkaloid), 32, 36, 38
Clitoris, 56
Clorox test, 85, 90-100; advantages, 100; procedure, 91, 100; reliability, 99, 100
Coca, 23-31, 32-9; alkaloids, 24, 25, 30, 31, 32-9; chewing, 23-4, 29, 31; and children, 23; as aphrodisiac, 24, 25; cocaine content, 29, 30, 31, 37; cultivation, 18, 25, 28, 30, 31, 40; description, 25, 29-31; legality, 29, 30, 31; and longevity, 24, 25; origin, 25, 29-31; processing, illicit, 33-7; production, 40; propagation, 25, 30, 31; species, 25, 29-31; vitamin content, 24, 54
Coca leaves, 12-13, 25, 29, 31, 38, 40, 71, 129-31; dry, to make pasta, 35, 41, 45; effects, 13-15, 24; odor, 29, 30
Cocaine abuse, 14-15, 47, 173-4, 179
Cocaine addiction, 48, 50, 173-4
Cocaine, adulterated. *See* Adulterants and adulteration; Cutting, of cocaine
Cocaine (alkaloid), 32, 33, 38, 52, 110; chemical

structure, 34; description, 38. *See also* Cocaine base
Cocaine and health, 47-62. *See also* specific effects and body parts
Cocaine base, 33, 36, 41, 45, 52, 56, 71, 76, 133-4, 140-1, 155, 160; amount needed to make cocaine, 45; and crystallization, 155-70; melting point, 74, 112; solubility, 89, 154
Cocaine base, converting to cocaine hydrochloride, 70-1, 155-6. *See also* Crystal labs; Crystallization
Cocaine base, pharmaceutical, 107
Cocaine base test, 110-22, 161; equipment, 111; procedure, 110, 114-22
"Cocaine bugs" phenomenon, 61
Cocaine, chronic use, 14, 48, 61
Cocaine color, 78-9
Cocaine cost, 44, 45, 62-3, 70; actual cost, 45, 146; equivalents, 62-3
Cocaine "crinkles," 139
Cocaine dependency, 14, 48
Cocaine, dirty, as deterrent to overuse, 155
Cocaine dosage, 13; frequency, 16
Cocaine effects, 11, 13-15, 38, 44, 47-53, 56-62, 74, 173-4; anesthetic, 14-15, 32, 37, 44; and ingestion method, 47-8
Cocaine etiquette, 78
Cocaine exporting, to U.S. and Europe, 42
Cocaine hydrochloride, 12, 13, 36-7, 41, 45, 52, 56, 79, 87, 95, 110, 133, 135-6, 155; crystallization, 155-70; melting point, 74, 104, 107, 142-3; solubility, 88, 89, 153, 154; tests, 113, 145
Cocaine hydrochloride, converting to cocaine base, 52, 155. *See also* Freebase
Cocaine hydrochloride, pharmaceutical. *See* Pharmaceutical cocaine
Cocaine ingestion methods, 15-16, 47-8, 50, 52, 56, 62. *See also* specific methods of ingestion
Cocaine Karma, 46
Cocaine laws, 25, 63-9
Cocaine market, 13, 17-19, 40-6, 70
Cocaine odor, 78. *See also* Wintergreen (odor)
Cocaine overdose, 18, 50, 51, 57, 179
Cocaine processing, illicit, 33-7, 155. *See also* "Cooks"; Kitchens; names of specific techniques
Cocaine purity, 12, 17-18, 70, 78-9; and color, 42, 78-9. *See also* Adulterants and adulteration
Cocaine, reinforcement by, 11, 14
Cocaine sulfate. *See* Pasta
Cocaine taste, 38, 79
Cocaine trade. *See* Cocaine market
Cocaine users, number of, 11-12, 179
Cocaine volume, 78-9
Coca-Cola, 25, 29, 30, 31
Cocamine (truxilline) (alkaloid), 32, 37-9, 78, 89, 107, 112, 134; effects, 37-8; taste, 38, 79
Coca wine, 25. *See also* Vin Mariani
Colombia, 25, 29, 30, 35, 36, 39, 41, 45, 71, 132, 134, 155
Color reaction test, 123
Connoisseurship, of cocaine use, 11-16, 54, 55, 156
Consumers (of cocaine), 11-16, 17-19, 43, 44, 45, 74, 78-9, 100, 179; and judgment, 15, 44, 48, 77, 123, 173
"Cooks," 33-7, 132, 134, 155, 157
Cost, of cocaine. *See* Cocaine cost
"Crashing," 48
"Crystal" (cocaine hydrochloride), 36, 45, 56. *See also* Cocaine hydrochloride
Crystal labs, 36-7, 41, 42, 45
Crystallization, 35, 36-7, 147, 149, 155-70; chemicals, 159; completion, 169; and cutting, 71; equipment, 158; procedure, 160-8
Crystals, of cocaine, 52, 86, 114, 170; drying, 168-70; growth, 157-69; washing, 169
Cutting, of cocaine, 13, 42, 45, 71, 74, 83, 100. *See also* Adulterants and adulteration; specific names of adulterants
Czar and Czarina (of Russia), 26

D

Dealer-users (of cocaine), 44, 45
Dealers (of cocaine), 43, 45, 46, 76-7, 100
Decantation, 149, 151, 166, 169. *See also* Acetone wash
Decomposition, of cocaine, 32, 34, 37, 39, 71, 78
Dehydration, 50, 54, 56
Depression, 48, 50, 173
Diet, 48, 50, 54
Diethyl ether. *See* Ether
Distributors, major (of cocaine), 42, 43, 45
Dr. McDope's Amazing Facts! (cartoon), 59
Doonesbury (cartoon), 58
Drug analysis labs, 15, 123-4, 175-7
Drug Enforcement Administration (DEA), 15, 124
Duff (powder), 78, 80-2, 87

E

Ecgonine, 32, 33, 34, 37, 38, 39, 71, 89, 107
Ecgonine conversion process, 33-7
Ecuador, 25, 30

Edison, Thomas, 26
Empanada, 136, 152, 167, 168, 169-70
Ephedrine, 89, 107
Erythroxylum coca, 25, 29, 30, 104, 129-31; cocaine content, 25; vitamin content, 54
Erythroxylum novogranatense, 29, 30, 31, 39; cocaine content, 29
Erythroxylum truxillense (var. of *E. novogranatense*), 30, 31, 37
Ethanol, 89-90
Ether, 36, 89-90, 133, 147, 155, 159; safety, 12. *See also* Petroleum ether
Ethyl acetate, 89-90
Exhaustion, 54
Extraction process, 52, 155. *See also* Cocaine base test

F

Farmers (of coca), 41, 45
"Fat Freddy's Cat" (cartoon), 49
Filter paper (in filtration and crystallization), 35, 136, 139, 149, 151, 152, 153, 167, 168, 170
Filtration, 35, 37, 52, 155, 156; gravity, 135, 149, 153, 169; vacuum, 133, 134
Flammarion, Camille, 26
Florida (port of entry), 42
Foil burn test, 42, 97, 101, 102-3, 144-5; procedure, 102-3
Forensic labs, 124-5
Freebase, 14, 52, 56, 58-62; dosage, 58, 60
Freebase smoking, 14, 15, 52, 54, 56, 58, 60; and health, 60-1; rush, 58, 60
Freebase snorting, 15
Freud, Sigmund, 62

G

Gasoline (as solvent), 35, 133
Gounod, Charles, 27
Guides (*guia*), 41, 45

H

Hallucinations, 15, 48, 60, 61
Health and cocaine use, 47-62. *See also* specific effects and body parts
Health centers directory, 179-90
Heart, effects from cocaine, 11, 14, 15; effects from freebase, 60
Heat lamp, 153, 167, 169-70
Huanaco coca. *See Erythroxylum coca*
Hydrochloric acid, 35, 36, 38-9, 71, 78, 133, 147, 153, 155-6, 159, 160-1
Hydrogen chloride, 159
Hygric acid, 38
Hygrine (alkaloid), 32, 36, 37, 38-9, 79, 89, 100, 107, 112, 113, 134, 137, 147
Hygrine hydrochloride, 89, 107, 153

I

The "impossible flake," 134
Impurities. *See* Adulterants and adulteration
Indians, South American, 13, 23, 24, 25
Inhalation, of cocaine, 48, 50, 54, 55, 157
Injection, of cocaine, 14, 15, 61-2
Inositol, 72, 73, 84, 89, 107; detection in tests, 72, 87, 88, 96, 99, 142-3, 144-5
Ipadu coca (var. of *E. coca*), 25, 29, 30

J

Java coca, 31, 32
Judgment, and cocaine, 15, 44, 48, 77, 123, 173

K

The "kind," 156, 157
Kitchens, 35, 41. *See also* "Cooks"

L

Laboratory testing, for cocaine, 123-5. *See also* Drug analysis labs
Lactose, 72, 73, 84, 107; detection in tests, 85, 87, 89, 95, 97, 99, 101, 142-3, 144-5
Lavigerie (cardinal), 27
Leo XIII (pope), 26, 27
Lidocaine, 14, 71, 73, 74, 83, 112; detection in tests, 98, 99, 122, 145; effects, 74
Lidocaine base, 85, 89, 98, 99, 107, 144-5
Lidocaine hydrochloride, 85, 89, 99, 107, 144-5
Lightweighting, 44, 46
Lilly pharmaceutical cocaine, 132
Lime, 23-4, 35
Longevity, and coca, 24, 25
Lungs, 15, 58, 60

M

Magnesium pemoline, 90, 107
Mama Coca, 22
Mannitol, 15, 71-2, 73, 83, 107; detection in tests, 85, 87, 90, 95, 97, 138, 142-3, 144-5
Mariani, Angelo, 25, 26-7

Marijuana, 18, 44, 54, 62
McKinley, William, 27
Melting point test, 85, 101, 104-9, 110, 138, 142-3; equipment, 105, 106-7; kits, 106-7; procedure, 104, 108-9
Melting points, 74, 101, 104, 106, 107, 112, 138, 142-3; of alkaloids, 38, 110
Merck pharmaceutical cocaine, 83, 86, 94, 132, 144-5
Methanol, 80, 161, 162, 163; as solvent, 89-90
Methanol solubility test, 87-8, 89-90
Methyl alcohol, 34, 37, 38
Methyl benzoate, 71, 80
Methyl benzoate test, 80, 113
Methyl salicylate, 29
Moisture, in cocaine, 79
"Moon disc," 135
Mother liquor, 149, 156, 166, 169
Mountain sickness, 13, 24

N

Nasal douche, 52, 55
Nicotine, 57
Nose care, 12, 52, 54-5, 147. *See also* Septum, perforated
Nose, effects from cocaine, 11, 12, 14, 15, 50, 52, 53, 147, 157; effects from adulterants, 14, 72, 147; effects from hydrochloric acid, 39, 147
Nose shape, after prolonged cocaine use, 52
Nosebleeds, 55

O

Operation Intercept, 18
Oral ingestion, of cocaine, 16, 62
Orgasms, 56
Overdose, of cocaine, 15, 50, 51, 57, 179
Oxidation process, 36

P

Paranoia, 15
Pasta (cocaine sulfate), 35, 36, 41, 45, 134; amount needed to make cocaine base, 45
Pasta labs, 35, 41, 45
Peanut butter craving, 54
Pearl cocaine, 139, 156, 157
Pemberton, John Styth, 25, 29
Pemoline, magnesium, 90, 107
Penis, 56
Peru, 23, 25, 27, 30, 31, 39, 41, 131
"Peruvian flake" cocaine, 83, 94, 132, 144-5
Petroleum ether, 52, 89-90, 134, 140, 141, 155; in cocaine base test, 113, 116-21
pH, of cocaine, 110, 112, 155, 156, 157, 159
Pharmaceutical cocaine (hydrochloride), 31, 32, 37, 83, 86, 94, 132, 144-5; melting point, 104, 107, 112
Phenylpropanolamine, 73, 74, 90, 100, 107
Pieces, of cocaine, 78, 80-2, 87
Potassium permanganate, 36
Potpourri (mixed-origin cocaine), 41, 42, 104, 112, 134
Procaine, 14, 74, 90, 107, 113
Psychogenetic dependency, 48
Purification, 146-70

Q

Quinine, 15, 72, 76; detection in tests, 87, 96, 144-5
Quinine sulfate, 85, 90, 107

R

Recrystallization, of freebase, 60
Rodin, Auguste, 27

S

Safety, 12, 56, 89, 110, 149, 153, 159
Sensory examination, of cocaine, 78-9
Septum, perforated, 14, 53, 55
Sex and cocaine, 56
Sheets (in crystallization), 35, 170
Smugglers (of cocaine), 42, 45
Snorting, of cocaine. *See* Inhalation, of cocaine
Sodium bicarbonate, 52
Sodium hydroxide, 80
Sodium hypochlorite, 90. *See also* Clorox test
Solubility, of cocaine, 87-90, 153, 154
Solubility tests, 76, 87-8
Solvents, 33, 35, 52, 87, 88, 89-90, 147, 149, 153, 155, 156, 157, 159; safety, 12, 56, 89, 110, 149, 153, 159
Sox, dirty, odor of, 38
Speed. *See* Amphetamine
Stirring, in crystallization, 161, 162-3
Stress, 14, 50, 54
Sucrose, 72, 90, 107
Sugar cut, 72, 78, 100, 101. *See also* Lactose; Sucrose
Sulfuric acid, 35, 36
Sun drying, of cocaine, 170

T

Talcum powder, 15
Testing kits, 77, 106-7
Tests, for cocaine, 72, 74, 76-145, 175. *See also* names of specific tests
Tetracaine, 74, 90, 107
Thin-layer chromatography, 124
Tolerance, of cocaine, 14
TOOT, 100
Treatment intervention, cocaine overdose, 51
Tropacocaine, 32, 38
ψ tropine, 38
Trujillo coca. *See Truxillense coca*
Truxillense coca (var. of *E. novogranatense*), 30, 31, 37
Truxillic acid, 37, 38

U

Urethra, 56

V

Vagina, 56
Venezuela, 29, 30, 71
Verne, Jules, 26, 27
Victoria (queen of England), 26
Vin Mariani, 25, 26-7
Vitamin consumption, when using cocaine, 50, 54
Vitamins, in coca leaves, 24, 54

W

Wash. *See* Acetone wash
Water, as solvent, 87
Water pipe (for freebase smoking), 52, 60, 141
Water solubility test, 87-8, 89-90
Wholesalers (of cocaine), 42, 45
Wintergreen (odor), 29, 39, 71, 78, 80
Withdrawal, from cocaine, 50, 173

Ordering Information

- Sorry, no COD orders. Prepayment in *US funds only* must accompany all orders.
- Add $1.00 for postage and handling. The order will be shipped to you via Special Fourth Class mail, or by surface post if you live overseas. Allow three to eight weeks for delivery. (Fourth Class mail is slow!)
- If you require faster delivery, please add the following *in addition to the above $1.00 fee:*
  First Class (USA and Canada): $1.00 per book.
  Air Mail (all other countries): $3.00 per book.
- Make check or money order payable to *What If?* for the total of the book(s) and postage charges. *Orders paid by personal check are held two weeks for bank clearance.*
- Be sure to include your name, address, and Zip code!
- Prices subject to change.

Order Form

Quantity	Title	Price	$19.95

☐ I live overseas and want my books sent Air Mail, so I'm enclosing an additional $3.00 per book.

☐ I want my books sent by 1st class mail, so I'm enclosing an additional $1.00 per book.

Subtotal ________

Postage ________

Amount ________

Enclosed is my ☐ check ☐ money order in US funds, payable to What If? for the Total amount.

NAME ________________

ADDRESS ________________

CITY/STATE/ZIP ________________

Send to: What If?, c/o Publishers Services, P.O. Box 3914, San Rafael, CA 94901